FOOD, NUTRITION AND HUNGER IN BANGLADESH

In fond memory of
Benjamin Halka Das

Food, Nutrition and Hunger
in Bangladesh

EDISON DAYAL

Avebury

Aldershot · Brookfield USA · Hong Kong · Singapore · Sydney

Published by
Avebury
Ashgate Publishing Ltd
Gower House
Croft Road
Aldershot
Hants GU11 3HR
England

Ashgate Publishing Company
Old Post Road
Brookfield
Vermont 05036
USA

British Library Cataloguing in Publication Data

Dayal, Edison
    Food, nutrition and hunger in Bangladesh
    1.Nutrition policy - Bangladesh 2.Hunger 3.Bangladesh -
    Social conditions
    I.Title
    363.8'095492

Library of Congress Catalog Card Number: 96-79946

ISBN 1 85972 582 1

Printed in Great Britain by
Antony Rowe Ltd, Chippenham, Wiltshire

Contents

Figures and tables

Preface

This book has grown out of my interest in the challenging problem of widespread hunger and undernutrition in Bangladesh. While teaching a course on 'Food, Nutrition, and Hunger: A Global Perspective', at the University of Wollongong, Australia, I collected much data and made three trips to Bangladesh to conduct field observations in 1985, 1988, and 1990.

Several researchers, who examined the food problem in Bangladesh in the 1970s and 1980s, presented a dismal picture for two reasons. First, they compared the situation in independent Bangladesh with that in East Pakistan. Such comparisons were based on data sets of different quality and reliability. Second, Bangladesh was grossly neglected under Pakistan, and the legacy continued well into the early 1970s. The analysis in this book is based on time series data from 1972-73 to 1991-92, which includes the period of most robust growth in Bangladesh. It uses both the national and regional scales to show the changes in food production and consumption. It shows that despite heavy odds, Bangladesh has made very impressive progress indeed in increasing food supply and reducing hunger and undernutrition. The evidence presented in the book indicates that food production has overtaken population growth; in fact the food situation in the country appears quite optimistic.

The book has 9 chapters. Chapters 1 and 2 are largely introductory and are based on compilations of information from a variety of sources. They are intended to provide a background for the understanding of the hunger problem in the country. Chapter 3 to 7 form the core and are based on original research. Chapter 3 presents a description of the agricultural scene. It examines the changes in the area of food and non-food crops and crop complexes over the two decades (1973-1992). Chapter 4 analyses trends in food supply and determines food production potential. Chapter 5 examines the impact of rapid population growth on food supply. The analysis in

xi

Chapters 6 and 7 examines food consumption levels and the extent of hunger. Chapter 8 reviews the role of government and non-government organizations in hunger alleviation, and Chapter 9 summarises the main ideas and makes some policy recommendations.

I am greatly indebted to Richard Miller for the final drafting of illustrations. Without his help it would have been impossible to meet the deadlines. I am also grateful to Dr. Stuart Pickering for reading the manuscript carefully and making many corrections and suggestions for improvement.

Finally, I am very grateful to my wife Dorothy for her support and encouragement throughout the writing of the book.

Edison Dayal
Wollongong
Australia   30 September 1996

1 Introduction

In the pre-colonial era, the area that is now occupied by Bangladesh was renowned for its productive agriculture, fine textiles, handicrafts, and general riches. Initially, the dense population of the Ganges delta must have been made possible by highly productive agriculture on very fertile land. Ibn Battuta, in his travels in north India, was most impressed by the economic prosperity of Bengal. The region that is now called Bangladesh was part of greater Bengal in undivided India. Battuta wrote,"This is a country of great extent, and one in which rice is extremely abundant. Indeed, I have seen no region on the earth where provisions are so plentiful" (Battuta 1958). Bernier (1891), a French traveller, who visited Bengal around 1660, was also amazed by the great variety of food and textiles. In his accounts, he described in some detail the great abundance of food at very low prices. Rice, vegetables of several kinds and butter were the common food of the ordinary people. He described Bengal as the storehouse of the finest cotton and silk, from where silk and cotton cloth were exported to Persia, Mesopotamia, Arabia, and even Europe and Japan. Bengal also exported rice, butter, and live animals to several countries. It was this abundance, he thought, that attracted people from all parts of the world into Bengal. Those who came never left. Several other writers have also presented a similar picture of 17th and 18th century Bengal (Chatfield 1808, Raychaudhuri 1953).

But now that image is tarnished by widespread poverty, hunger, and malnutrition. The country is now characterised by its high population densities, large agricultural work force toiling on innumerable small holdings producing rice, heavy dependence on foreign aid, and general political discontent. In its short history as an independent nation, it has had several military coups and assassinations of political leaders. The official statistics portray a trend of declining hunger and malnutrition, but a recent UNICEF report reveals a dismal picture (UNICEF 1995). The report reveals that unlike most other nations of the world, where the average height of people has been increasing due to improved nutrition,

1

the average height in Bangladesh has been declining due to increased malnutrition. The report states that 90 percent of the children under 2 years of age are stunted. By international standards, only 7 percent of the children under two years may be considered normal in height and weight for age. This may be true because the food and nutrition situation began to improve only recently and it may take some time before the improvements begin to show in the health and demographic variables.

Implications of hunger for development

Hunger and undernutrition are cruel because they impede development and deprive a society of some basic comforts of life. They have devastating effects on human physical health and intellect. Several medical problems such as xerophthalmia, goitre, and anaemia , to mention only a few, are caused by nutritional deficiencies. Poor health and disease impair learning abilities of children and prevent the development of their full potential, resulting in a lower level of skills acquired. For example, marasmus results in a reduced number of brain cells (Warnock 1987, Robinson 1978). Also, inadequate intake of food or undernutrition results in stunted growth of body and consequently in low productivity and incomes (Dutra de Oliveira et al 1985). It is quite understandable that people having small body size and low weight are disadvantaged in several spheres of physical activity (Dasgupta and Ray 1990). Available evidence, therefore, shows that undernourished people remain physically and intellectually underdeveloped and are invariably in lower socio-economic classes. Undernourishment, in general, has an adverse effect on the quality of human resources and has a negative impact on development. Dasgupta and Ray (1986) have shown that unemployment is linked to the incidence of malnutrition. They suggest that short-run programs of employment generation must necessarily involve food transfers.

A glimpse into the history of hunger in Bangladesh

The history of hunger in Bangladesh is unclear. The few accounts bearing on the economic history of the region that are available for the 16th, 17th, and 18th centuries have not made clear-cut statements on the extent of hunger (Hunter 1875, Habib 1963). There is some mention of the rich and poor households, but it is hard to guess how poor the poor households were. It is not clear whether they suffered from food poverty or were simply relatively poor. But from the accounts of Ibn Battuta and Bernier, it appears that even the poor were adequately fed. Hunter (1875) describes the quality of food intake for the business households and peasant households. The food of a peasant household was very similar to that of a business household, except that it was coarser in quality. Habib (1963) reports that there were landless agricultural labourers in Bengal in the 16th century, when the population would have been quite small. Although unused land that could be occupied by any landless members of the society was available, the members of the depressed classes still cultivated the land that belonged to others. They were discriminated against and

2

could never aspire to become peasants. They had the legal right to occupy unused land but they were prevented from doing so by the more powerful members of the society, who acted in their own interests. This implies that land was sufficient in quantity. There is no mention of the quantity and quality of food consumed by the landless agricultural households. However, Habib stated that cultivating classes were better off, just as they continue to be today in rural Bangladesh. Perhaps the relative poverty always existed in Bangladesh as elsewhere in the world but widespread food poverty became more apparent in the present century. Nevertheless, even up to 1947 Bangladesh was self-sufficient in food supply (Hossain 1980).

The environment of hunger

The persistence of hunger in a given region is often due to a variety of reasons, but gross inequality in the distribution of land and income is the paramount reason. Some people remain hungry because they lack the power to purchase adequate food. Persistent hunger, therefore, is the outcome of the prevailing social, economic, and political systems that widen the gap between the rich and the poor. Such systems may operate at all levels — international, national, and local— and deny to some people the basic right to food (Bennet 1987, Warnock 1987). But the poor in Bangladesh, as elsewhere in the world, are so powerless that they can do nothing to modify the system.

Although it is widely held that hunger is man-made, adverse natural environments often aggravate the situation. For example, those who normally manage to feed themselves but are at the economic margin often slip down into the category of the hungry when crops fail due to some aspect of weather or climate.

The physical environment

An acute shortage of food-producing land imposes very serious limitations on adequate food production. It is probably the second most important cause of hunger and undernutrition in Bangladesh after inequality in the distribution of wealth. The total area of the country is only about 55,000 sq. miles (144,000 sq. km), of which about 15 percent is occupied by rivers, ponds, and other non-agricultural uses. Consequently, the land-people ratio (0.5) is one of the lowest in the world. Because the population is still growing quite rapidly, the land-people ratio is consistently declining. Between 1971 and 1991, it dropped by 29 percent. The possibilities of bringing more land under food production are almost nil. Several economic historians have stated that the scope for the expansion of agricultural land had been exhausted in Bengal as early as the 17th century. The shortage of land is so acute that people use every bit of land and even temporary river islands (*chars*), which have a short life of only a couple of years, are used for cultivation. Therefore, increased food supply in Bangladesh must come from a practically constant input of land.

The quality of land resources is good. The agricultural land is very fertile and its

3

fertility is annually renewed by new sediments laid over it by flood waters. Despite the high fertility of the land, per acre yields of crops were among the lowest in Asia, until recently (Hossain and Jones 1983). But they increased very significantly in the 1980s, and now stand above many countries in Asia and Africa.

Water resources are plentiful, but they must be tamed to be of use for increasing food output through irrigation expansion. In 1995, about 33 percent of the total cropped area in Bangladesh was irrigated, and Bangladesh was among the 20 top countries in terms of net irrigated area. There is ample scope and also need for expanding irrigated area in order to boost food production in the dry winter season.

The climate of Bangladesh is both good and bad for crop production. It is good because temperatures are high enough to permit year-round cultivation. It is bad because the distribution of rainfall is so uneven that in the summer months heavy rains accompanied by the rush of water from the north cause deep floods over large areas, inflicting heavy damage to crops, and in winter the soil moisture is not sufficient for most crops except in some low lying areas. The rainfall is heavily concentrated in the few monsoon months, leaving the rest of the year dry.

Bangladesh is also one of the most disaster-prone countries in the world. Frequent floods, cyclones, and droughts do considerable damage to food crops and aggravate the problems of hunger and malnutrition in the country. The natural hazards are responsible for wide fluctuations in food supply. Often the drop in food supply is so large that the country is compelled to import large quantities of foodgrains and even ask for food aid. The extent of hunger and undernutrition escalates whenever a major disaster hits the country, and that is not infrequent. The impact of natural hazards on the lives of the people was beautifully described in the *New York Times* a few years ago. "Life in the shadow of disasters has bred a race of tough, fierce men and women. Their very existence on those shores depends on their being ferocious" (*New York Times*, June 21, 1987).

The social and political environments

Causes of hunger are many and complex. Hunger is often the result of past policies and projects such as the replacement of traditional food production systems by modern market-oriented systems. These two kinds of system are very different in character. The primary objective of the traditional food production systems was to provide food for the peasantry, but that of the new market-oriented system is to make profit, even if it may mean replacement of food crops by export crops. In the pre-colonial era, agricultural production was largely to produce food for the growers and for some others in the local areas who provided various services to the farmers. The replacement of food crops by cash crops began to reduce local food supplies, and made farmers dependent on others for their food supply. The gradual expansion of cash crops led to a large number of small producers and only a few buyers. The buyers were local agents of foreign companies. Therefore, the producers had no control over the market price of cash crops. Often, over-supply reduced the price of cash crops below the local food prices and farmers began to be affected by hunger. Further, the introduction of death control but not birth control, and discouragement of manufacturing, escalated hunger in the countries that were previously colonies of European powers. These policies led to faster growth of population, reduction in domestic food supply, landlessness, and lack of employment opportunities in manufacturing (where increased population could have been transferred), and aggravation of hunger in Bangladesh as in other European colonies.

The British destroyed the economy of Bengal, first by destroying the cotton textile industry, and second by destroying agriculture. The Bengal textiles were disallowed entry into Britain, and were also discriminated against within India by the tax system imposed. A silky variety of cotton had been grown in Bengal from which the famous Dacca muslin was made (Datta 1936). That variety has now become totally extinct. In Bengal, the British destroyed agriculture by rapid expansion of area under cash crops such as tobacco, cotton, sugarcane, indigo, and jute, all for the British mills. The planters advanced credit to the peasant farmers and then compelled them to grow the crop they wanted. This led to a system of quasi-forced labour (Grigg 1974). Continued cultivation of cash crops, some of which were very demanding on soils, accelerated soil erosion. The crop yields began to decline and so did the incomes of cultivators. Further, the introduction of the zamindari system had a damaging effect on agriculture and particularly on food production. Before the British, the zamindars were simply collectors of taxes for the Moughal state. The British made them owners of land. Thereafter, the zamindars began to exploit the peasants, which destroyed their incentive to increase production and had a negative effect on food supply. Hence the colonies became more and more dependent on industrial countries for the supply of not only industrial goods but also food. They assumed a subordinate role of supplying raw materials and some food to the European industrial powers. Interference with an agricultural system that was geared to producing food for the local populations, the misuse of land, and the introduction of unsuitable tenure systems laid the foundation for the escalation of hunger in Bengal.

The exploitation of Bangladesh by West Pakistan was, perhaps, even worse than that by the British and led to a further increase in hunger and poverty. The extent of hunger became worse in the 1950s and 1960s, when the region was part of Pakistan. During that period there was unmistakable exploitation of Bangladesh on the colonial pattern. The economic policy was so designed that it encouraged industrial development of the west at the expense of the east. Further, it was designed to keep the eastern wing as a captive market for the industrial goods produced in the west. The discriminatory pattern of development is evidenced by the allocation of development funds between the two wings of the country. In the First Five Year Plan of Pakistan, 80 percent of the development funds were invested in the west. In the subsequent plans, the allocation of funds for the eastern wing improved a little but not much. In the Third Plan, which ended just before the birth of Bangladesh, the western wing was again allocated 64 percent of the development funds despite the fact that more than half the population of Pakistan was in the east

(Chowdhury 1972). In the 1950s and 1960s most of the foreign exchange was earned by exporting jute and jute products from East Pakistan, but it was all used for the development of the West. Also, the bulk of the foreign aid, including food aid, was spent on the west (Ayoob et al 1971). As a result of this discriminatory treatment, the per capita incomes in 1970 were 61 percent higher in the west, but prices of food were 150 to 200 percent higher in the East. Hence, there was a much greater concentration of hunger and poverty in the Bangladesh region. The underdevelopment and poverty, created by the discriminatory economic policy of West Pakistan, continued well into the 1970s in Bangladesh. After becoming independent, Bangladesh had to start the development process almost from scratch. Hence, an analysis of change based on a comparison of undifferentiated pre-independence and post-independence data is likely to be misleading. The war of liberation also did considerable damage to agriculture and disrupted food supply. After the war, it took a year for the supply to reach the pre-war level. The whole countryside was terrorised by the patrolling army. The supply of seed and fertilizers was interrupted. The labourers, both males and females, were reluctant to work in the fields for fear of being taken for forced labour by the army. A number of roads, bridges, irrigation channels and embankments were destroyed by the army in order to stop the advancement of the Indian army.

Far too often the causes of hunger outlined above are not given enough weight, and attention is focused only on population size and inadequate supply of arable land as the main causes of hunger. During the last 50 years the food supply in the world has increased as never before despite the more than doubling of the world population. Food supply has surpassed population growth but in several countries hunger has increased. In 1988, the number of hungry in the world was estimated to be 600 million, roughly 12 percent of the world population (Kates et al 1988).

In Bangladesh, between 1971 and 1991, the population increased by 46.6 percent but rice production increased by 80 percent, thus surpassing population growth. Despite faster growth of production than population, hunger and undernutrition still persist. The major cause of hunger in Bangladesh is very high inequality in the distribution of income and land resources. Inadequate employment opportunities in both rural and urban areas also contribute to the creation of hunger. Whenever there is a shortage of food, the landless and underemployed lose their entitlement first. This happens because as soon as a natural calamity — a flood, a cyclone, a drought or a crop disease — gives a signal for a forthcoming food shortage, the big farmers begin to hoard foodgrains in order to create artificial scarcity for the purpose of raising food prices. The landless agricultural labourers, artisans, and small farmers have no surplus to hoard. If the food production really drops, the demand for their labour also drops, eroding their food-purchasing power. Hence, they begin to suffer from hunger.

The existing levels of hunger and malnutrition in Bangladesh are not due to inadequate supply of food but due to maldistribution of available resources. In this respect, the situation in Bangladesh is similar to that in the rest of the world. In Bangladesh, 10 percent of the rural households own 50 percent of the agricultural

6

land. About 60 percent of the households own the remaining half, and about 30 percent are landless. The landless households are the poorest and suffer considerably from hunger and malnutrition. They are suppressed, exploited, and made to work on very low wages. For example, in Bangladesh, the landless have the legal right to occupy *char* land — temporary islands in the rivers — which appears at several locations after the flood waters recede. But the rich landowners, who enjoy formidable power in the rural society, by using the power and labour at their disposal, occupy this land before the landless can. They make the landless work on this land for low wages for their own gain. Thus, the landless, instead of being the owners of *char* land, end up cultivating it for the rich landowners. They recently formed an action group to fight for their legal right to acquire *char* land, but were confronted by very strong opposition from the rich landlords, who have been trying to crush the movement by using all unfair and illegal means within their power.

It is indeed commendable that despite heavy odds — severe scarcity of arable land, the large and fast growing population, high inequality in the ownership of food producing resources, and the very high frequency of natural disasters, all of which resist efforts to increase food production — Bangladesh has managed to bring down the incidence of hunger and food poverty considerably. On the basis of 2,122 calories per person as the minimum daily requirement, the level of food poverty dropped from 83 percent in 1973-74 to 48 percent in 1991-92. Now the level of hunger and undernutrition in Bangladesh is not much higher than in other countries of South Asia. This has happened practically without any change in income distribution (BBS 1995). The efforts that are now being made to reduce income inequality through employment generation must further reduce hunger in the 1990s.

Is population a major cause of hunger?

In 1991, 111 million people were crammed into about 36 million acres of land. This gives an average density of 3 persons per acre of total area or 5.24 persons per acre of net cropped area. These are unusually high densities of population and make Bangladesh three times more densely populated than India and seven times more densely populated than China. The distribution of population is fairly uniform, but the eastern and central districts are more densely populated. The most densely populated districts are Chittagong, Comilla, Noakhali, and Dhaka, where the densities of population on both total and net cropped area are well above the average for Bangladesh. The western districts along the Indian border are generally less densely populated. Chittagong HT, Patuakhali, and Dinajpur have the lowest population densities. There is no doubt that a large population on a small area exerts severe constraints on the supply of land for food production in Bangladesh. However, Hayami and Ruttan (1985) have shown that even in a situation like this the potential for agricultural growth still exists, which can be realised by increasing technical inputs and human capital. In fact this has been amply demonstrated in Bangladesh as we shall see later.

Until recently, high population densities and growth were regarded as the main

7

causes of poverty and hunger. It was assumed that more people consume more and produce relatively less. But this idea began to lose support when several densely populated countries began to record enormous increases in food production soon after the end of the colonial era. For example, Japan, Taiwan, and Korea, with 50 times more agricultural workers on agricultural land than the USA, produce more food per hectare than the USA. Even China, with 250 times more agricultural workers on agricultural land than the USA, is not far behind the USA in food output per hectare. Bangladesh today has more agricultural workers per unit of land than India, Pakistan, the Philippines, and Thailand, but it produces more food per hectare than any of them. Similarly, it produces considerably more food per acre than most of the African countries, despite much heavier population pressure on land. There is no doubt that a large and rapidly increasing population puts more strain on the food production system but at the same time it increases the possibility of food production efficiency (Simon 1983). This has been demonstrated by Bangladesh and several other Asian countries. During colonial times, most farmers did not have much access to markets, therefore they only produced what they could consume or sell in the local markets. Because the populations were small and most people produced their own food, the demands in the local markets were small. Since the end of the colonial era, the populations in most countries of Asia have increased but the total food intake of people has also improved. Hence, it is now widely held that high population densities and growth are not the main cause of hunger. Several studies have confirmed that there is no correlation between hunger and population density (Foster 1992, Uvin 1994).

This does not mean that population is not causing any problems. The government recognizes that large and rapidly growing population will delay the achievement of self-sufficiency in food. Therefore, it is taking positive measures to control population growth. Bangladesh is one of the very few Muslim countries where population control has been seriously undertaken, and where it is beginning to show results. Between 1974 and 1991, the exponential growth rate per year, total fertility, and crude birth rate per thousand dropped from 2.48 to 2.17, 6.34 to 4.18, and 40 to 30 respectively. The mean age of females at marriage increased from 15.9 to 18.1 years, and the number of females getting married between the ages of 10 and 14 dropped by 41 percent during the period. These are important changes indeed and clearly show that the government is concerned about high population growth and seriously doing something about it. The government effort to curb the growth of population will certainly improve food supply per capita and help further reduce hunger in the country. Much of the success has come from doorstep family planning, which employs more than 23,000 women to distribute contraceptives and advise women about the benefits of smaller families. The government realises that for a successful population control program the social status of women must be lifted. Therefore, 15 percent of the public sector jobs are currently reserved for women.

A rapidly growing population demands large investment in education for even maintaining a certain level of abilities and skills of population. The level of education has a positive effect on skills acquired and consequently on income and food intake (Knight and Sabot 1987). For a rapidly growing population a large investment is required for training more teachers, building more schools and colleges, printing and improving more text books, and providing more school transport etc. The slowing down of population growth in Bangladesh appears to be helping the improvement of its level of education and skills. Between 1974 and 1991, two population census years, the population increased by 60 percent, but the number of teachers increased by 128 percent and the number of students by 218 percent. These figures could be misleading because they do not show growth in population of persons of school-going age; nevertheless, they do show that the expansion of educational facilities is keeping pace with population growth.

Prospects for eliminating hunger

When Bangladesh became independent, about 80 percent of its population was inadequately fed. Now the level is much lower because the eradication of hunger and poverty have received a high priority in development planning in independent Bangladesh. Also, Bangladesh has been greatly helped towards the achievement of this goal by large amounts of foreign monetary aid, direct food aid, and project food aid. Although Bangladesh now produces enough food to satisfy effective demand, considerable hunger and malnutrition still exist. Nevertheless, important progress in hunger reduction has been made and is continuing. For example, in the Fourth Plan, which ended in 1995, more than a quarter of the total outlay of the plan was for the development of agriculture, water resources, and other rural infrastructure to help increase food production. In the Fourth Plan, special emphasis is placed on increasing the production of pulses, maize, fruits, and vegetables, besides rice and wheat. As increased production alone is not very effective in eliminating hunger and malnutrition, the Fourth Plan also focuses on the growth of national income through industrialisation and expansion of employment opportunities. More work opportunities will enable poor households, who cannot afford to buy enough food now, to improve their food intake. Increased food production and purchasing power are rightly expected to eradicate hunger and malnutrition in the country. However, the country will have to overcome formidable difficulties in achieving the goal. First of all, the land resources for food production are limited and there is no scope for their expansion. Hence, increased food output must come from increased productivity. Although there is good scope for this at present, it cannot go on indefinitely. Nevertheless, very impressive progress in this direction has also been made since independence.

Increased production and population control are two essential but not sufficient requirements for the eradication of hunger, malnutrition, and poverty in Bangladesh. It is also essential to transfer population from agriculture to non-agricultural activities, i.e., manufacturing and service industries. However, in Bangladesh, resource endowment for manufacturing at present is very poor. There are practically no minerals, no oil, no forests, and no coal. But there is enormous manpower, which can be profitably used in manufacturing based on imported raw materials, particularly for labour intensive industries that need only a low level of technology. There is sufficient scope for the development of labour intensive industries such as food processing, textiles, footwear, and clothing. Once the necessary skills for manufacturing have developed in the work force, further industrialsation can depend on imported raw materials. Considerable efforts are being made to expand and diversify manufacturing in order to increase job opportunities and improve the balance of trade position. Several manufacturing industries are now developing with the collaboration of foreign partners, but some entirely by national entrepreneurs. Labour intensive industries such as jute and cotton textiles, food processing, and leather tanning emerged first to take advantage of the cheap labour. Textile, clothing, and food manufacturing are the top three manufacturing industries, and the next three are industrial chemicals, iron and steel , and leather goods. Engineering, steel re-rolling, and fertilizer industries are also important. Textile, clothing, jute products, leather goods, and even electrical appliances are now exported to Europe and other developed economic regions, and are earning desperately needed foreign exchange. Bangladesh now has a positive balance of trade with Europe, but has a negative balance with Asia, the Middle East, and Australia. The development of manufacturing will have important indirect effects on the reduction of hunger and food poverty. It will reduce unemployment and underemployment by creating more work opportunities in both rural and urban regions, reduce pressure on agricultural land, and increase labour productivity and incomes. Further, the development of manufacturing will increase the country's foreign exchange earnings and enhance the food purchasing power of the nation and also of the individuals. Development of manufacturing in recent years has not only improved the balance of payment position but has also led to the expansion of services and is now beginning to change the structure of the national economy. In 1992-93, agriculture contributed only 33 percent to the GDP, services contributed 57 percent, and manufacturing 10 percent. However, agriculture is still very important in the national economy as it produces a variety of food and cash crops and employs 61 percent of the labour force.

Food imports and food aid have both helped in reducing hunger. Bangladesh continues to receive food aid from several countries and the UN. In 1992, the country received $US 241 million worth of food aid in the form of grants. Bangladesh does not take food aid loans any more, because the domestic food supply has increased considerably. In times of natural calamities though, food aid is still required. If the supply continues to increase as it has in the late 1980s and early 1990s, there is no doubt that Bangladesh will soon be able to build sufficient reserve stocks even for emergencies. Although food aid is very helpful, it often does not reach those who need it most. There is considerable mismanagement and corruption in handling food aid. A large proportion of food aid is distributed to government employees through ration shops, and only a little of it goes to the rural poor.

The large and increasing negative balance of trade is a major economic problem which has serious implications for hunger. In 1991-92, the negative balance of trade stood at 57 billion takas. Without the remittances by Bangladeshi nationals and non-nationals living overseas, and international grants and aids, the situation would have been quite hopeless. Often the remittances are more than the aid. The negative balance of trade greatly limits the scope for importing various food items that may continue to be important for improving the quality of diet and adding more variety to it. The problem of inadequate foreign exchange for buying some food from outside is likely to persist for quite some time. Hence, the drive towards food self-sufficiency is a move in the right direction.

Looking at the progress of Bangladesh since independence, one feels optimistic about the reduction of hunger. The progress on all the fronts that may reduce hunger and malnutrition, i.e., food supply, food distribution, population control, employment opportunities, and trade balance, appears to be very significant. Although Bangladesh is much less fortunate than India in respect of per capita resources and is more prone to natural disasters, it is not far behind in the reduction of hunger and malnutrition.

What this book is about

Using empirical data, this study sets out to explore how independent Bangladesh has tackled the problem of feeding its large and increasing population and reducing hunger over a twenty-year period (1972-73 to 1992-93). The analysis presented in the book investigates several interrelated questions about food, nutrition, and hunger in Bangladesh. How have the farmers reacted to increasing food demand in the country ? What has been the impact of population growth and consequent increase in food demand on the cropping pattern, frequency of cultivation, methods of food production, and government food policy? How much food can Bangladesh produce and how stable is the supply? How have the food consumption standards changed over time? What is the extent of hunger and how has it changed over time? How effective has government policy been in increasing food supply and protecting food exchange entitlement of the poor? These are important questions that must be examined into in order to understand the hunger problem in the country.

The demand for food is a major variable that determines the productive efforts of farmers and changes production methods and crop pattern. Hence, one of our concerns is to identify the changes in the cropping pattern and methods of production. In the situation that prevails in Bangladesh, farmers can only increase food production by increasing the level of land-augmenting inputs (irrigation, fertilizers, insecticides, and HYV seeds) and or the frequency of cultivation. Both the available alternatives increase output per acre. The growing demand for food has had a positive influence on the cropping pattern and methods of production. The cropping pattern has been changing in favour of high yielding food crops and those that are less vulnerable to natural hazards. It has been noted that the area under each main variety of rice has increased but that under *Boro* increased most. Wheat, a relatively new crop, is now making a significant contribution to the reduction of

11

hunger. The analysis of trends clearly shows that, contrary to general belief, food production has consistently increased, despite decreasing land resources, increasing population pressure on land, and vagaries of climate. Besides foodgrains, the output of fruits, vegetables, meat, and fish has also increased considerably. It will be shown that the domestic production of ten major food crops can provide more than 2,000 calories for each consumption unit. Using a simple but rigorous objective method to calculate the food production potential in Bangladesh, we will show that the food supply in Bangladesh can be further increased by at least 30 percent, using known technology and plant breeds.

There is unmistakable evidence that agricultural intensification — both in terms of frequency of cultivation and levels of inputs — has continued to increase along with rapidly increasing labour force. In some densely populated regions, food production intensity has reached a near maximum. Hence, we noted a regional shift in the intensification of food production from more densely populated to less densely populated regions. To explain this process, we will examine the growth of food production, cropping intensity, and population in Bangladesh and its districts over time, and develop a new regional theory of agricultural intensification.

Using household expenditure data and also Bangladesh Bureau of Statistics (BBS) data, we have explored how the nutritional value of the average diet as well as diet in all income groups has changed. We have also examined how the extent of hunger has changed and what factors are responsible for the change.

The Government policy is clearly in favour of increasing food supply in order to gain the favour of the urban elites because they exercise considerable influence on the masses. The government is committed to achieving self-sufficiency in food supply and reducing hunger. To do this the government has invested heavily in the expansion of irrigation, flood control, new agricultural technology, rural infrastructure, agricultural research, and food entitlement protection. In these ventures the government has been helped immensely by non-government organizations. These policies are proving effective in reducing hunger.

To further reduce the level of hunger, more determined efforts will have to be made to protect food entitlements of the poor. At present government policy favours the urbanites but the majority of the hungry live in the rural areas. Policies to provide price support and security of tenure to small farmers, and more effective policies to reduce concentration of land ownership will further reduce hunger in Bangladesh.

The data and their reliability

The analysis of food production and hunger in this book is based entirely on official food production and consumption statistics, collected and published by the Bangladesh Bureau of Statistics. Several researchers have questioned the reliability of Bangladesh data for acreage and production of crops, because the data were for a long time based on highly subjective methods of estimate (Boyce 1987, Pray 1980, Alauddin and Tisdell 1987). The Department of Agriculture collected acreage and production data through its extension staff, who estimated the acreage and yield rates of a crop by interviewing selected local farmers and by their own observations. The information so collected was compared with the estimates of previous years and with those obtained in the 1944-45 plot to plot survey — a comprehensive enumeration undertaken by the Government of Bengal. How exactly the 1944-45 enumeration influenced the annual figures in subsequent years was not clearly revealed. Similarly, the annual estimates of the yield per acre were influenced by the 'normal' yield, which was again a vague concept. In practice, therefore, the subjective estimates were rightly considered unreliable by users.

To improve the reliability of acreage and production figures, the Department of Agriculture in undivided Pakistan introduced the objective method of estimation. The method is based on a stratified random sample of a number of 5 acre plots in each district. There are now 5753 sample clusters that are used for the estimation of area and yield per acre of major crops (GOB 1987). These plots are carefully examined for land use and crop acreages. The percentage of area under each crop in the plots is then used for the estimation of crop acreage in the districts. For estimating the yield per acre, crop cutting surveys are conducted during the harvesting seasons of different crops. These experiments are conducted on a sub-sample of plots in the clusters by well trained field staff of the Bureau of Statistics and also by the *thana* (smallest civil division) and district agricultural officers. Initially, the crop cuts were conducted on rectangular areas (1/80 of an acre) but in 1979-80 more efficient circular cuts were introduced and subsequently extended throughout the country. The field staff remains in close touch with the operators of sample plots and seek their cooperation in conducting crop cutting surveys. For determining the dry weight of the crop, 500 grams of green paddy or other grains are sun dried by the BBS field staff until the weight of the sample stabilizes. The production figures are obtained by multiplying estimated area by yield per acre for each district.

The official data for crop acreages and production have improved immensely since the introduction of objective methods of estimation based on crop cutting surveys on randomly selected sample plots. By the mid 1960s, the entire country was covered by the objective methods of estimation of area and production of all major crops. However, the system was disrupted in 1971, during the war of liberation, and in the following year because of changes in responsibility for data collection. From 1973 onwards, the data seem to have become quite reliable due to refinements in methods of collection, better coverage of area and crops, and better training of field staff. Some studies based on farm level data, collected by the authors, found that the results of their analysis were consistent with those based on official district statistics (Hossain 1974). Such studies have confirmed the reliability of data after the mid 1960s. Soon after the country gained independence, the Bangladesh Bureau of Statistics launched a serious program to improve further the accuracy of agricultural data. They introduced more comprehensive training including more advanced techniques of measurement for the field staff, and they also increased the numbers of field staff. Further, they initiated a scheme of checking the activities of the field staff by senior officers without notifying field staff in advance. Therefore, since independence the accuracy of data has improved even more. However, one runs into problems when using long time series data extending back beyond the mid 1960s. In doing that, one has to use data collected by two very different methods and hence of different quality. Obviously, the results of the analysis based on data of different quality and reliability are bound to be dubious, if careful adjustments are not made, which is often very difficult. In this study, therefore, to analyse changes in food supply we have used data only for independent Bangladesh. It is believed that changes revealed for independent Bangladesh are least affected by changes in the quality of data. Also, to exclude the effects of interruptions in agricultural activities and data collection during 1971 and 1972, these two years were dropped from the time series or not included in the base period. To minimize the effects of minor fluctuations that are due to weather, three year averages were taken to assess changes in acreage and production. Also, agriculture, like all other economic development, was grossly neglected in Bangladesh when it was a part of Pakistan. To compare the state of agriculture then with the present is unfair, as it is bound to exaggerate changes.

Food consumption data seem to be more reliable because they are collected in household surveys by actually contacting the consumers. There are two sources of food consumption data. The first is the Household Expenditure Survey which is conducted on a large sample — around 12,000 households — and covers expenditure on about 1,500 items. The expenditure on food items is carefully recorded for the past one week. The expenditure data are, therefore, a reliable source for calculating the quantity of nutrients consumed by individuals and households and have been extensively used for estimating food poverty in Bangladesh and other south Asian countries. The second source of consumption data is the National Nutrition Survey, which is based on a smaller sample — about 700 households — but has the advantage of providing information on actual quantities of food consumed. Every item of food consumed in the household is weighed and carefully recorded. Hence, even food items collected free for consumption are taken into account. Therefore, Nutrition Surveys give more accurate consumption data. In this study, we have used Household Expenditure survey data because they are available for a longer period and also for more recent years.

Nutrition policy

Food policy in Bangladesh must be focused on reducing inequality in the distribution of land and other sources of income, and creating more employment opportunities for the landless and small cultivators. This will increase the purchasing power of the poor.

The government's efforts to redistribute land through land reform measures have not been very successful. Some scholars, however, consider that land reform measures are not going to help in the agrarian situation that now prevails in Bangladesh, because there is simply not much land locked up in large holdings that will make a substantial difference if redistributed. The number of holdings larger than 10 hectares is very small. Therefore, more attention should be focused on lifting the food purchasing power of the landless households and tenant farmers without redistribution of land. This can be done by promoting capital works programs and creating other non-agricultural employment opportunities in rural areas. The government is already directing attention in this direction through the introduction of Food for Works Program (FWP). This program is part of a much wider Public Food Distribution System (PFDS), which is operational in Bangladesh to fight food poverty. The program is believed to be quite effective in reducing hunger and malnutrition among those who participate in it and also the members of their households. The Fourth Five Year Plan (1990-95) has been particularly focused on increasing productive employment and thereby lifting the food entitlement of the poor. The other measures to increase access to food for the poor households are price control and distribution of foodgrains at subsidised prices through ration shops. However, food rationing does not necessarily help the poor households because ration cards are issued on the basis of residential status and not on income. Now the emphasis appears to be shifting from subsidized food rationing to the PFDS.

Another important area to which the government must direct attention is improving the condition of the tenant farmers by providing more security of tenure and a greater share of the output. This will provide them with the incentive to produce more. Not much appears to have been done in this direction. Tenant farmers are still very much at the mercy of the landlords.

Finally, development of manufacturing and service sectors in a land-scarce economy is crucial. It will have multiple benefits. First, it will help transfer some population from agriculture and reduce population pressure on land, which may assist in raising labour productivity. Second, it may increase the purchasing power of wage workers, both in rural and urban areas. Third, it will generate more foreign exchange by reducing imports of some manufactured goods and by increasing exports of some other manufactures. Fourth, the expansion of manufacturing will also attract foreign investment which will accelerate economic growth. All the above developments will have a positive impact on the nutritional status of the people.

Summary

During the pre-colonial period there was little or no hunger in the region now called Bangladesh. Hunger began to escalate during the colonial period and reached a peak just before the region became an independent country in 1971. The major causes of hunger in Bangladesh are an acute shortage of land, very high inequality in the distribution of land resources and income, landlessness, inadequate employment opportunities in the rural areas, and frequent destruction of crops and even reserve stocks by natural hazards.

An attempt will be made to examine how independent Bangladesh has tackled the problem of feeding its growing population from the meagre land resources available. Between 1972 and 1992 food production surpassed population growth; and now there are real prospects of reducing hunger to the level of the Asian average.

2 Resource endowment for food production

Increasing food supply in a given region is limited not only by the size and quality of physical resources, but also by social, economic, and political constraints. Despite increasing application of science to the production and processing of food, the food production industry is and will continue to be predominantly resource based. The size and quality of physical resources can both be adversely affected by human activities. For example, the size and quality of land resources in Bangladesh appears to be diminishing due to over use of land in agriculture, expansion of non-agricultural uses of land, land tenure policy, and destruction of natural vegetation, which are contributing to rapid erosion and loss of fertility of agricultural land. Crop yields would have dropped considerably if fertilizer use had not increased over time. In Bangladesh, land and climatic resources impose the most serious constraints on food production, and this is one area in which the government can do little to improve the situation.

Agricultural land, water resources, and climate

Plants need warmth, moisture, sunshine, and soil nutrients for their growth. The regions with a better combination of these are more favourable for food production. For example, in some regions, winters may be too cold and long and may allow crop production only for a few months in a year. In some others, summers may be too hot and dry for plant growth. The physical environment may often impose serious limitations on food production. This section, therefore, presents a brief account of the major characteristics of the physical environment of Bangladesh.

Land

The size and quality of land are the most important endowment of a nation, because

17

they are the source of all wealth. In an agrarian economy, like Bangladesh, where land is the main source of livelihood for over 80 percent of its population, the importance of land cannot be over-emphasized. If we ignore capital and organization, which are both relatively unimportant in traditional food production systems, then land and labour are the two major factors of production. Land is a physical resource, and its supply is fixed by the land area of a nation. As a physical resource, it is considered indestructible by economists (Barlowe 1972). But as an economic resource, its supply is a function of demand. Its supply for a given use can be increased, if people agree to pay the additional cost of land development. Therefore many economists believe that there is no shortage of land (Crosson 1982, Raup 1982). Perhaps it was this view that led to a widespread squandering of land resources in the world. The sooner we realize that land is not simply a commodity that can be used indefinitely without giving it any rest and replenishment for producing goods, the better it will be for the survival of mankind. Land is much more than an economic commodity, since it plays an important role as a link in the maze of life. As the quantity of land is fixed, it is one of the most sought after resource. It has been looked upon, generally, with reverence in the past and continues to be so treated at least in some societies. Several major wars have been fought for gaining possession of land. The present economic prosperity of nations like the U.S.A., Canada, and Australia may be attributed to a variety of factors, but it may not be completely wrong to say that it is partly due to the large land resources they possess (Barlowe 1972).

The position of Bangladesh with respect to land resources is very unfortunate. The total area of Bangladesh is 55,598 sq. miles (143,998 sq. km), and is fixed, but the population is still increasing quite rapidly at the annual rate of 2.2 percent in recent years. A significant proportion of the total area is occupied by more than 200 major rivers and their tributaries, which criss-cross the low plains of Bangladesh (Figure 2.1). About 15 percent of the total area is occupied by rivers, settlements, and irrigation tanks. Hence, the actual area available for agricultural use is only 134,476 sq. km, much less than the total area. Consequently, the land-man ratio is very low, 0.50 acres (0.2 Hc) and continually declining. For the arable land, the land-man ratio is only 0.30 acres (0.12 Hc). With this ratio it is almost impossible for Bangladesh to be self-sufficient in food supply, except through very intensive use of land. The land-man ratio in Bangladesh is worse than in most agrarian economies of Asia (Table 2.1). Undoubtedly, therefore, the resource base for food production is very limited in relation to the size of its population. This also explains why a high proportion of potentially arable land is effective land in Bangladesh. "Land is real hunger in Bangladesh, therefore, sixty percent of the population is landless" (Cobb Jr 1993).

In some countries there is no scarcity of land, but much of the land is of little economic value, as for example in Australia and several African countries, because either it is not used for production at all or it is used too extensively. But in Bangladesh, all land is scarce relative to population, therefore everywhere it is used

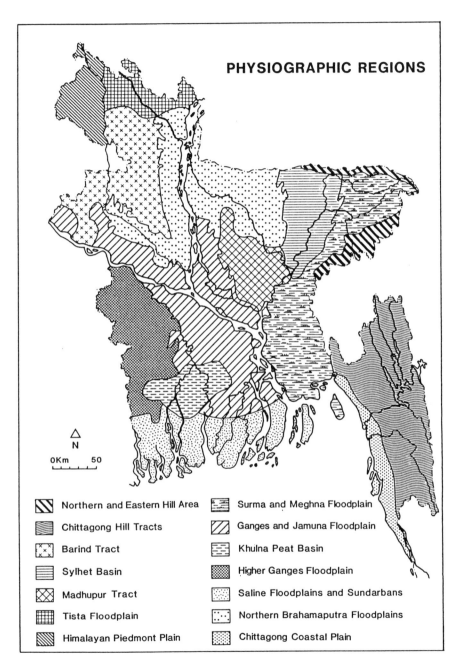

PHYSIOGRAPHIC REGIONS

N

0 Km 50

Northern and Eastern Hill Area		Surma and Meghna Floodplain	
Chittagong Hill Tracts		Ganges and Jamuna Floodplain	
Barind Tract		Khulna Peat Basin	
Sylhet Basin		Higher Ganges Floodplain	
Madhupur Tract		Saline Floodplains and Sundarbans	
Tista Floodplain		Northern Brahamaputra Floodplains	
Himalayan Piedmont Plain		Chittagong Coastal Plain	

Figure 2.1 Physiographic regions of Bangladesh

19

very intensively. At present 64 percent of the total area is under cultivation. The remaining area is either not usable for agriculture or is under non-agricultural uses.

Increasing population pressure continues to compel people to bring additional land under cultivation. Therefore, despite little scope for expansion of agricultural land, it increased by 800,000 acres or at the rate of 40,000 acres per year, which is hardly 0.04 percent, between 1971-72 and 1990-91. Therefore, practically there was little change in cultivated area. As land began to be cultivated more intensively to

Table 2.1
Land-people ratios in selected Asian countries in 1992

Countries	Arable land	Population total	agricultural	Land-people ratio total pop.	agricultural pop.
	(000 Hc)	(000)	(000)		
India	165,400	772,106	495,371	0.214	0.333
China	97,373	1,072,079	753,185	0.091	0.129
Japan	4,209	121,492	9,295	0.035	0.453
Indonesia	15,500	169,356	81,089	0.091	0.191
Bangladesh	8,866	103,821	73,833	0.085	0.120

Source: Calculated by the author from FAO data

meet increasing demand for food, it also began to lose its fertility more rapidly. Apparently it became necessary to leave more land under current and long fallow as reflected in Figure 2.2 and Table 2.2. The net cropped area per head of rural population and also per head of male agricultural worker has been consistently declining (Table 2.3). The net cropped area per head of rural population declined by 29 percent between 1974 and 1991 and per head of male agricultural workers by 40 percent. These figures clearly demonstrate the seriousness of the problem of land shortage in Bangladesh and how it is deteriorating over time.

The possibilities of expansion of agricultural land are so lean that the proportion of total area which is cultivated has remained nearly constant over the last 50 years (Islam 1978). In some regions the cultivated land even declined. It is possible that some land must have become marginal due to over use and therefore abandoned. Some has been taken up by shifting of river channels. The major rivers of Bangladesh are known to carry enormous load of sediments. Being in their old age, the hydraulic efficiency of rivers is low. As their strength to carry the load is further reduced during the low flow, they drop much of the sand and gravel on the channel floor. Such depositions cause the rivers to shift sideways towards the lower ground. The lateral shifting of rivers in any one season may be over a distance of up to 300 metres. The lateral advances along the river banks may be up to 850 metres in a single year (Brammer 1993). Hence, over a period of time large areas are lost to agriculture by lateral shifting of river channels in Bangladesh. The Brahmaputra river has, for example, shifted about 113 kilometres to the west in the last 200 years. This regular, but unpredictable, shifting of the massive rivers results in devastating loss of agricultural land, human settlements and activities. In 1988, the Meghna river changed its course and cut a new channel 120 feet deep (Cobb Jr. 1993). Some arable land is annually taken up by expanding rural and urban settlements. In densely populated villages in Bangladesh 3 to 4 percent of the land is taken up by dwellings, roads, footpaths, and embankments (Arnon and Isaac 1987).

Table 2.2
Land use trends in Bangladesh

(Million acres)

Years	Net cropped area	Current fallow	Long fallow	Cultivated area
1971-72	20.4	2.1	0.7	23.2
1972-73	20.8	1.7	0.7	23.2
1973-74	21.0	1.5	0.7	23.2
1974-75	20.6	2.0	0.7	23.3
1975-76	21.0	1.6	0.7	23.3
1976-77	20.4	2.1	0.7	23.2
1977-78	20.7	1.8	0.7	23.2
1978-79	20.8	1.8	0.6	23.2
1979-80	20.9	1.7	0.6	23.2
1980-81	21.2	1.4	0.6	23.2
1981-82	21.2	1.3	0.6	23.1
1982-83	21.4	1.2	0.6	23.2
1983-84	21.4	1.1	0.8	23.3
1984-85	21.3	1.2	0.7	23.2
1985-86	21.7	1.0	0.7	23.4
1986-87	21.9	1.0	0.6	24.3
1987-88	20.5	2.9	0.9	24.3
1988-89	20.1	3.3	0.9	24.3
1989-90	20.6	2.7	0.9	24.2
1990-91	20.2	2.4	1.4	24.0

Source: Agricultural Yearbook of Bangladesh, various issues
Note: Cultivated area = Net Cropped Area + Current Fallow + Long Fallow

The scarcity of land is so acute that despite the risk of complete submergence and consequent destruction of crops during the floods, even the small river islands and several areas prone to deep annual flooding are used for food production. In some years, the cultivators may be lucky and may get a good output from such areas but in other years the crop may be entirely lost due to complete submergence under flood waters. However, water has the power to destroy land and also to create it. In Bangladesh, while valuable cropland is annually lost by erosion of river banks and sheet erosion during floods, a number of *chars* are also created every year by the deposition of silt transported by rivers. *Chars* are temporary islands because they disappear within a few years. But even during their short span of life they are used intensively by land hungry peasants. Cobb Jr. (1993) reported 475 families living on a *char*, only 2,000 feet long and 70 feet wide. Such areas produce at least one good crop during the winter season.

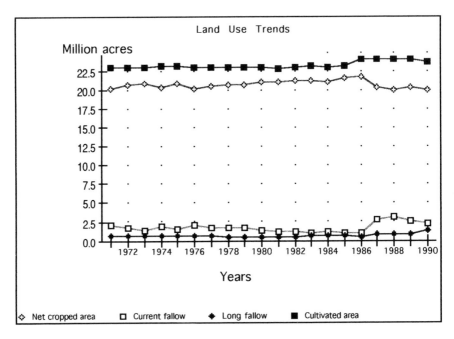

Figure 2.2   Land use trends in Bangladesh

Various estimates have been made about the potential arable land for different regions of the world. Even for Asia, about 20 percent of the non-arable land is reported to be arable by some researchers. But no such optimistic statement appears possible for Bangladesh because of unceasing efforts to expand cultivation throughout the 18th, 19th, and 20th centuries. By the end of the 19th century, cultivation had already extended to even the most marginal lands to produce cheap inferior crops for the poor (Kelly 1981). There is also evidence that application of manure on the rice crop began in 1870s, indicating that expansion of crops on new

22

land was becoming difficult. Under such conditions, the priorities in the allocation of land to various uses are much more critical than in sparsely populated regions. Further, the population pressure is so great that the human population, in an effort to survive, may destroy the rare and irreplaceable ecosystem, because they know of no other alternatives.

Table 2.3
Per capita net cropped area for selected years

Years	Rural population	Male agricultural workers
1973-74	0.318	1.10
1980-81	0.243	0.99
1984-85	*	0.91
1990-91	0.225	0.65

Note: Total number of agricultural workers over time are not comparable because of changes in the definition of female workers. Therefore, only male agricultural workers are taken.
* Data not available
Source: Calculated by the author from BBS data

Although the area used for cropping has remained more or less constant, the area under multiple cropping has been steadily increasing. The area under multiple cropping appears to have increased because of increase in the irrigated area and introduction of High Yielding Rice Varieties (HYRVs). The HYRVs are short duration crops; therefore they have been instrumental in the expansion of winter rice and wheat. The HYRVs are harvested earlier than traditional varieties and give more time for the cultivation of a second or third crop on the same land. The pattern and form of land use usually change in response to growing population, because additional people have to be accommodated on the same land. The intensity of cultivation increases and the cropping pattern changes in favour of food crops. This is exactly what has been happening in Bangladesh during the last two decades at least.

Survival and prosperity of human society depend not only on the quantity of land but also on its quality. Much of the land in Bangladesh, having been built by the tertiary sediments brought down by the mighty Ganga-Padma, Brahmaputra-Jamuna, and Meghna river systems, is very fertile. As the eastern Himalayas and the

Shillong Plateau receive heavy rainfall during the monsoon, the river systems carry enormous loads of sediments, which have formed the plains of Bangladesh. The thickness of the sediments is unknown. Ganga and Brahmaputra bring more than two million tons of suspended material daily (Spate and Learmonth 1967). Much of this material is dropped either in Bangladesh or in the Bay of Bengal. Borings have reached depths of more than 1,300 feet without hitting the bed-rock (Johnson 1975). More then 80 percent of the area of the country is flat, and it rises very gently towards the north and the northeast, but nowhere is the elevation more than 80 feet above sea level, excluding the hills. Sylhet, which is about 250 miles inland, is only 48 feet above sea level. The southern districts of Bangladesh are at sea level. Therefore, global warming due to the increasing CO_2 level in the atmosphere, resulting in sea level rise, is of special concern to Bangladesh. A two to three feet rise in sea level, which is expected by the middle of next century (Chiras 1991), may submerge large areas in Bangladesh. This may help one to understand the problem of floods that cover large areas annually and are devastating for agriculture in some years.

The deposits which constitute the plains are of Pleistocene and more recent origin. The older deposits have been uplifted at certain locations, where they are locally called *bhanger* . They are generally 18 to 40 feet above the flood plains. In the east and southeast, there are the Chittagong Hills with an average height of 2,000 feet. In the north, the Dinajpur and Rangpur districts are occupied by piedmont alluvial plains. The rest of the country is an extensive, flat, and fertile alluvial plain. The fertility of these plains is annually renewed by the fresh silt, nitrogen-fixing algae, and decomposed plants spread over land during the floods. For this reason, some writers have described Bangladesh as the most fertile region of the world. It is ironic that such an area should be so poor and so dependent on others for food. Obviously it is the extremely adverse man-land ratio and frequent natural calamities that explain at least part of the situation.

Sylhet and western parts of Mymensing comprise the Sylhet basin the lowest area in Bangladesh. This entire area is flooded every year during the monsoons, when rivers overflow their banks (Umitsu 1993). Over this large tract farming during the monsoon period is, therefore, very restricted. About two thirds of the massive delta of the Ganga and Brahmaputra occupies the southern one third of the country (Figure 2.1). In the delta region the relief is much less pronounced. The distributories often cross the interfluves and create a checkerboard pattern of river systems. The fluvial activities produce perpetual changes in the morphology of the delta region. The regional allocation of land to crops is significantly affected by the minor relief differences that exist in the otherwise flat plains. *Aus* rice and grain legumes occupy the highest land, jute the middle slopes, and winter *Boro* rice the lowest area, which often retains more soil moisture for winter crops.

About a third of the total area of Bangladesh is subjected to deep flooding in summers, and hence is often not available for *Aman* crop. This area lies mainly in the centre, along the Padma, Jamuna, and Brahamputra, but also in the Sylhet Basin in the east. After excluding these areas that are either not available for agriculture or where agriculture stands a high risk, the area available for reliable crop production is indeed small. Therefore, about half the holdings are less than 2.5 acres.

The soils of Bangladesh have been variously classified by different writers. Broadly, they may be classified into three main groups, i.e., hill soils, alluvial soils, and swamp soils. Almost 90 percent of the land area is alluvium (BBS 1992). The alluvial soils are divided into two main groups as calcareous and non-calcareous. The soils in each of these two groups are further differentiated on the basis of the colour of the alluvium, i.e., gray, dark gray, and brown. Sometimes the alluvial soils are divided into five categories on the basis of their geographic location, e.g., Brahmaputra alluvium, Ganga alluvium, Teesta silt, Madhopur Tract, Barind Tracts (Figure 2.1). These sub-categories indicate the river system from which they have been derived. The Madhopur and Barind Tracts both consist of relatively older quasi-lateritic alluviums, and stand higher than the surrounding alluvial deposits in the form of terraces (Spate and Learmonth 1967). They occupy the central and northwestern parts of Bangladesh. The soil in Madhopur Tract is red clayey laterite; it is rich in iron and alluminium. In the Barind Tract, soils are brownish in colour and poor in nitrogen, phosphorus, and lime. The Bramhaputra alluvium occupies approximately the north central part of the country, where its continuity is interrupted by the outcrop of Madhopur Tracts. The Ganga alluvium occupies the southwestern parts, and Teesta alluvium the northern. The hill soils are found in the Chittagong hills and in the foothills along the northern border. The swamp soils occupy the delta region and are also known as saline tracts. They are clayey and reasonably rich in humus.

The soils of Bangladesh have been derived from the tertiary rocks, Pleistocene sediments, and recent deposits. Each of these parent materials has produced a distinct soil type. All the new alluvial soils are very similar in character. They contain adequately high levels of potassium oxides and lime, but are generally poor in nitrogen and humus. The deficiency of nitrogen is more pronounced in the western districts of Kushtia, Jessore, Pabna, and Rajshahi.

There are significant regional variations in the structure of alluvial soils in terms of grain size and porosity. Generally, soils close to the major rivers are sandy and gravelly. They are coarse and too porous for rice cultivation, but are still used. They get too dry during winters and considerably reduce possibilities of multiple cropping. Large tracts of such soils are found in the Faridpur, Rangpur, and Dinajpur districts. Further, sizable tracts in Faridpur and a few other southern districts consist of peat and muck. They remain permanently wet and can be used for only one crop of broadcast *Aman* rice.

Further, in the southern districts of Khulna, Patuakhali, Barisal, and Coastal Noakhali there are large areas where the soils suffer from high salinity, which is due to inland penetration of salt water through tidal waves. Much of the land in this tract is new. Soils are relatively rich in potash and phosphate. They cover a large area of about 6,000sq. miles.

The soils in Bangladesh are generally fertile. The silt that forms the various alluvial soils is derived from a variety of rocks, and is therefore rich in mineral salts. The fertility of the soils is annually replenished by fresh silt spread over arable land. Therefore, the soils have continued to produce reasonably good yields without the use of much fertilizer. Bramer (1990) has disputed the general belief that fresh silt brought down by rivers and spread in the fields by flood waters is fertile and improves productivity. He argues that fresh silt becomes fertile after several years. There is, however, no doubt that the fertility of the soil after the floods improves, but probably it is from nitrogen-fixing blue-green algae living in the water and from the decomposing of submerged plants and animals.

Structure and distribution of agricultural holdings

The 1983-84 *Census of Agriculture* is the most accurate and reliable source of information on the number and size distribution of agricultural holdings in Bangladesh. In the census year, 73 percent of the households were farm households, who were operating more than 0.04 acres of cultivated area. The farm households operate a very high proportion (96%) of farmland they own. The non-farm households, on the other hand, operate less than 40 percent of the farmland they own. This is because non-farm houesholds lease out their land to farm households for operation, because it is too small for cultivation.

The pattern of farm holdings in Bangladesh is heavily dominated by small farms. More than 70 percent of the farms are small farms, being less than 2.49 acres. The medium and large farms are 25 and 5 percent of all farms respectively (Table 2.4). Although the small farms dominate the scene, they account for less than a third of the farmland, only a little more than the farmland area occupied by large farms.

The distribution pattern of farm holdings is quite distinct as it clearly shows the regional concentration of small and large farms. The largest concentration of small farms appears to be in the southeastern and central districts, where, on an average, 80 percent of the farms are small. There appears to be a regional accord in the concentration of small farms and high population density (Table 2.5). For example, in Chittagong, Comilla, Noakhali, and Dhaka, the most densely populated districts of Bangladesh, small farms account for more than 40 percent of the farmland.

The percentage of farmland in medium sized farms (2.5 -7.5 ac) appears to be fairly uniform across districts, except in the hilly districts. In most districts, medium sized farms account for 45 to 50 percent of the farmland. The large farms are clearly concentrated in the less densely populated districts all along the western boundary. In addition to the western districts there is also some concentration of large farms in the hill districts in the east.

The ownership pattern of farm holdings is highly skewed. The top 10 percent of the largest farm owners own about half the farmland. To make matter worse, the degree of concentration of land ownership seems to be increasing over time (Jannuzi and Peach 1980, Banik 1990, Ahmad 1987). Landlessness has been commonly explained in terms of rapidly increasing population, but this is not supported by empirical evidence. For example, the percentage of households having no land was the highest in Dinajpur and Rangpur, which are certainly not the most densely populated districts in Bangladesh. On the other hand, the lowest percentage of landless households is in the most densely populated districts of Comilla and Noakhali. Thus, the regional distribution of landlessness in Bangladesh confirms the view that population density does not have any significant impact on landlessness (BBS 1986). The most important reason perhaps is that land is still considered a valuable asset and a secure investment. Therefore, big landlords, who have money, continue to invest in land. Whenever a piece of land comes into market the big landowners grab it, even though they do not cultivate all their existing land themselves.

Table 2.4
Size distribution of farm holdings

Size of farms (acres)	Percentage of farm numbers		Percentage of farm area	
	1977	1983-84	1977	1983-84
< 0.5 *	*5.47*	*24.06*	*0.50*	*2.74*
Small farms (<2.5)	49.72	70.34	18.75	28.98
Medium farms (<7.5)	40.85	24.72	48.90	45.09
Large farms (> 7.5)	9.40	4.92	32.36	25.92
All farm households	100.00	100.00	100.00	100.00

Note: * Percentages in italics are for the smallest farms, which are already included in the percentages of the small farm category.
Source: Compiled from the data in The Bangladesh Census of Agriculture 1983-84

Jannuzi and Peach (1980) estimated that half the households in Bangladesh were functionally landless because they owned less than 0.5 acre, excluding homestead land. The 1983-84 census gives a much lower level of functionally landless farm households (24%).

27

Table 2.5
Percentage of small farms and rural population density on net cropped area

Districts	Percentage of small farms 1983-84	Rural population per acre 1981
Chittagong HT	45.6	2.64
Chittagong	79.8	4.32
Comilla	84.4	4.32
Noakhali	83.4	3.42
Sylhet	67.1	2.66
Dhaka	78.9	4.28
Faridpur	70.5	3.31
Jamalpur	69.7	2.92
Mymensingh	69.8	2.92
Tangil	72.3	3.45
Barisal	75.6	3.21
Jessore	59.1	2.54
Khulna	66.2	3.10
Kushita	62.3	2.84
Patuakhali	66.7	2.28
Bogra	71.1	3.02
Dinajpur	51.4	2.20
Pabna	64.8	3.29
Rajshahi	60.3	2.44
Rangpur	67.2	3.12
BANGLADESH	70.3	3.11

Source: Calculated by the author from BBS data

It is interesting to note that despite a high degree of concentration of land ownership, the incidence of tenancy in Bangladesh is not very high. Less than 10 percent of all farm households are purely tenant households. But the percentage of owner-cum-tenant farmers, who cultivate their own land as well as some land of others, is quite high (around 35%). This level of tenancy in Bangladesh has remained strikingly stable despite rapid rural population growth and increasing concentration of ownership of farmland. There is, however, considerable regional variation in the incidence of tenancy. The tenant and owner-cum-tenant farmers, who cultivate small areas, generally less than two acres, are clearly more concentrated in the Chittagong, Dinajpur, and Rajshahi districts. Their lowest concentration is in the Khulna and Sylhet districts. The tenant and owner-cum-tenant farmers cultivate small areas because they cannot raise capital for buying inputs. They either have no assets to mortgage or have very little, and therefore banks are generally unwilling to give them credit.

The most common type of tenancy in Bangladesh is share-cropping, and the most prevalent arrangement is that the tenant supplies all the inputs required for cultivation. The whole burden of supplying labour and inputs falls on the tenant farmer but his share of the output is the same as that of the landowner. There are no written contracts, therefore tenant farmers do not remain on the same land for very long. In most cases they are evicted after a few years. This is done to ensure that they do not make any claim over the land, if the government adopts a policy of land to the tiller.

Significant changes have occurred in the agrarian structure of Bangladesh over time that were examined by Banik (1990) for the period between 1960 and 1984. During this period the number of households in the smallest farm size category increased by 123 percent and the net cultivated area in this category increased by 89 percent. Because all farm households and the net cultivated area increased only by 64 and 65 percent respectively, it may be inferred that the rest of the increase in both was due to transfer from other categories. This is confirmed by the changes in both the number of households and cultivated area in the large farm size category, where they declined by 24 and 28 percent respectively. The percentage of all households in the small size category increased from 52 in 1960 to 70 in 1984 leading to a significant decline in cultivated land per head. The annual rate of increase for small farm households was 2.7 percent. On the other hand, the percentage of farm households in the large size category dropped from 38 to 26, at the annual rate of 0.2 percent. This is one indication of increased concentration of large farms in fewer lands. The increased concentration of land ownership is further confirmed by the gini coefficient, which increased from 0.5008 to 0.5477 during the period.

Banik (1990) provides three explanations for the changes hat have occurred in the agrarian structure of Bangladesh during the 25 year period. The increase in the number of small farm-households has certainly been affected by population growth and laws of inheritance that have led to subdivision and fragmentation of farm holdings. The gradual disintegration of the rural joint family system may also have contributed to the growth of small farms. Further, it is possible that some landowners in the medium and large category who became wealthy acquired more land from other categories.

The pattern of change in the agrarian structure that is leading to an increase in the number of small holdings and their fragmentation is a matter of serious concern. But some scholars have argued that in the situation prevailing in Bangladesh, small farms will not impede food supply. Small farms have several advantages. They provide more employment for the large and increasing labour force and more equitable distribution of income, and they enable more households to depend on their own production rather than becoming landless labourers. In a labour surplus less mechanized economy, the productivity per unit of land has been found to be consistently higher on small farms (Hossain 1977, Sen 1964, Khusroo 1964, Steven and Jabara 1988). High land productivity on small farms is achieved by using high input of family labour that results in a very low marginal productivity of labour (Desai and Majumdar 1970, Mellor and Stevens 1965, Sen 1960). But low marginal productivity of labour in the context of Bangladesh and other densely populated land scarce regions is not considered a serious disadvantage as long as the average product of labour is greater than or equal to the subsistence level. However, if the farms continue to become smaller and smaller, a point will be reached when the average product of labour will be less than the subsistence level, and that will lead to an increase in hunger and starvation.

Fragmentation of farms is posing an equally serious problem that may have a negative impact on food supply. About 70 percent of all agricultural holdings have fragments ranging from 4 to 10. Sometimes they are several kilometres apart. A fragmented holding is more expensive to operate and is also wasteful of time and effort.

The unsatisfactory agrarian structure can be sometimes corrected by taking some land reform measures. The problems of land reform in Bangladesh will be discussed in Chapter 8. Here I will only making a passing comment on the ongoing debate concerning land reform in Bangladesh. It is widely believed that land reform leading to redistribution of land in Bangladesh will create insurmountable difficulties and may not significantly change the existing situation (Hussain 1989). Perhaps, redistribution of land is neither possible nor very effective in improving the present situation, but certainly something can be done to deal with fragmentation of holdings and also to improve the conditions of tenant farmers. For example, the consolidation of holdings, which has proved very successful in increasing productivity in several countries of Europe and India, can also be implemented in Bangladesh. Also, tenant farming can be made more attractive by providing greater security of tenure to the tenant farmers, and by introducing legislation for more equitable distribution of gains and responsibilities between tenants and landowners. For example, if the landowners want half the share of the output they should also make some contribution to the inputs. At present they contribute only land, which is only one of the many inputs required for crop production. Therefore, it is only fair that the tenant farmer gets a larger share of the output. Both these changes — consolidation of holdings and improvements in tenancy legislation — may certainly be expected to have a positive impact on food supply in Bangladesh.

Water resources

Bangladesh is a well watered area. There is no lack of surface or underground water resources for the development of irrigation for food production. The country is criss-crossed by innumerable streams, and possesses a large reservoir of underground water. Further, the natural rainfall is quite plentiful, and the need for irrigation, during most of the year, is not large. Irrigation is needed in relatively higher areas largely for winter crops. Highly seasonal concentration of annual rainfall makes expansion of irrigation quite important for raising output of winter crops through multiple cropping.

During the winter season only about 20 percent of the net cropped area is cultivated, although temperatures are ideal for the cultivation of several crops such as *Boro* rice, wheat, barley, potatoes, several grain legumes, and oil seeds. In winter, only a few months after the monsoon rains stop, the lack of moisture in the soil does not permit the utilization of about 80 percent of the fertile, newly silted arable land. Therefore, expansion of suitable irrigation can increase multiple cropping quite considerably in Bangladesh, and change it from a food deficit to a food surplus country. For this reason expansion of irrigation has received a good deal of priority in development planning since Bangladesh became independent. However, at present less than 30 percent of the net cropped area is irrigated. At the end of the Third Five Year Plan, which ended in 1990, total irrigated area was 7.5 million acres, which was 31 percent of cultivated land. But the emphasis on increasing it further continued in the Fourth Plan as indicated by the allocation of funds for the development of water resources. The increase in the irrigated area since independence has been quite impressive. Between 1970-71 and 1990-91 the net irrigated area increased from 3 to 7.5 million acres, an increase of 150 percent (Table 2.6). During the same period the area irrigated by tube-wells increased by a staggering 4,300 percent. The area irrigated by tube-wells increased from 0.1 million acres to 4.4 million acres in a period of about 20 years (Table 2.6). As canal irrigation is not suitable for a wet country like Bangladesh, its expansion appears to have received low priority. Expansion of canal irrigation is likely to cause waterlogging problems as the water table in Bangladesh is quite high, and will also further reduce surface area now available for cultivation. Nevertheless, canal irrigation, during the same period, increased also by 100 percent.

There is plenty of surface water in Bangladesh during the monsoon season, but much of it goes to waste into the sea. It carries with it millions of tons of very fertile sediments that can be used for improving fertility of the existing land or building new land if prevented from being dumped into the sea and lost forever. If even a small fraction of this water could be stored for use during the dry winter season, it would certainly help increase food production and supply much needed fertile soil for a variety of uses. Of course it is easier said than done, but it is not impossible. A novel scheme for the storage of more surface water has been presented in the following paragraph

Increasing the area under conventional tanks to store surface water will take too much of the valuable cropland of which there is already an acute scarcity. However, it is possible to increase the storage capacity of existing tanks that are located in the areas subject to deep flooding or near the river banks, without taking any new land. This may be done by building reinforced concrete tanks protruding vertically upward to an appropriate height, which may be several thousand feet above ground.

Table 2.6
Changes in irrigated area by methods

Irrigation type	1972-73 (000 ac)	1990-91 (000 ac)	Percentage change
Power pumps	1,165	1,667	43.1
Tube-wells	93	4,404	4,635.5
Canals	236	427	80.9
Others	1,499	980	34.6
TOTAL	2,993	7,478	149.8

Source: Calculated by the author from BBS data

During the monsoon season, excess water will have to be pumped for storage into these vertical tanks, and would be released during the dry winter for irrigation. Some energy will be required for lifting water, periodic cleaning of tanks, and for manipulation of gates, but releasing water for irrigation will need no energy, because it will depend on the force of gravity. These tanks, of course, will soon be filled with the most fertile and valuable sediments brought in suspended form with the water. But that should not cause insurmountable problems. In fact the collection of fertile sediments will be an advantage rather than a drawback. The bottom end of the tank could be provided with manoeuvrable gates, similar to those installed in irrigation dams. These gates could be used for extracting sediments at regular intervals. The best time for extracting sediments would be the end of the winter season when there will be little or no water left in the tank. The labour costs of cleaning tanks may be more than recovered by selling the fertile sediments for a variety of uses. There is always a ready market for soil in Bangladesh for making nursery beds, spreading over fields, repairing field embankments, making raised ground for building houses, making bricks etc. Yet another advantage of the scheme will be a reduction in the area under deep flooding during the monsoon season because excess water will be pumped up for storage in the tanks. Hence, some more land will become available for food crops.

The suggested scheme sounds entirely feasible. The technology required for the construction of vertical tanks is already available and is practised widely in Bangladesh. For example, lifting water by electric or oil pumps is a common practice in rice farming. Also, all along the coast thousands of reinforced concrete structures have been built by the government and by non-government organizations for use as cyclone shelters. Hence, the construction of vertical tanks is not likely to pose any serious technological problems. The only environmental problem that one can think of, is that the seepage of water that may raise the water table. But this can be easily overcome by making the bottom of the tank impervious.

Climate

Bangladesh enjoys a warm and humid sub-tropical climate. The average monthly temperatures are high enough to permit year round crop production. The average monthly maximum temperatures in winter are around 27.5 C (80 F), and the minimum well over 10.0 C (50 F) providing frost free seasons for cropping. The difference between winter and summer temperatures is not large. The average summer maximum temperature is 37 C. Hence, moisture supply becomes the main constraint for crop production in some months of the year. The pattern and rhythm of human activities in Bangladesh, as in the rest of the sub-continent, are dominated by the monsoon rains. The hopes and fears of the peasant, and indeed of the whole economy, hang on the timing and the amount of monsoon rains in a given year.

The annual average rainfall in Bangladesh is 2,546 mm. Its variations across districts are not strikingly large except in Sylhet. Also, there is a narrow strip of land in the west-central part of the country, which is the driest. It gets an annual average rainfall of 1,500 mm (Figure 2.3). In Rajshahi, which gets minimum rain, the average is 66 percent of the mean for all districts. Hence, no region of Bangladesh appears to be seriously disadvantaged for agriculture due to lack of soil moisture during the monsoon season. Sylhet and Chittagong districts, being on the windward side of the mountain ranges, take the full onslaught of monsoon winds and receive maximum rainfall. Sylhet is located just south of Cherrapunji - the rainiest place on earth. It gets twice as much rain as Dhaka. The rice crop needs roughly 50 mm of rain per month (Johnson 1975). The annual average rainfall would be more than the minimum need for rice crop as prescribed by Johnson, if only it was uniformly distributed over the year.

Although the annual average rainfall (2,546 mm) is a lot more than adequate for agriculture, its distribution over time, as already said, is very uneven. A great bulk of the annual rain comes during the four monsoon months of June to September, which account for about 80 percent of the annual total (Table 2.7). During the months of December to March, soil moisture is inadequate for plant growth, except in some low lying areas, where accumulation of monsoon flood water keeps soil moisture at a higher level for a longer period. Such areas have sufficient soil moisture in winters for several crops such as wheat, gram, peas, and oil seeds; but elsewhere irrigation is required to grow winter crops (*Rabi*). This seasonal variability of rain is a major encumbrance in increasing food production in Bangladesh.

The annual variability of rainfall, as one would expect in a high rainfall region, is low, being less than 15 percent, but in some regions it may reach 20 percent above or below normal. But variability of annual rainfall is really not important in

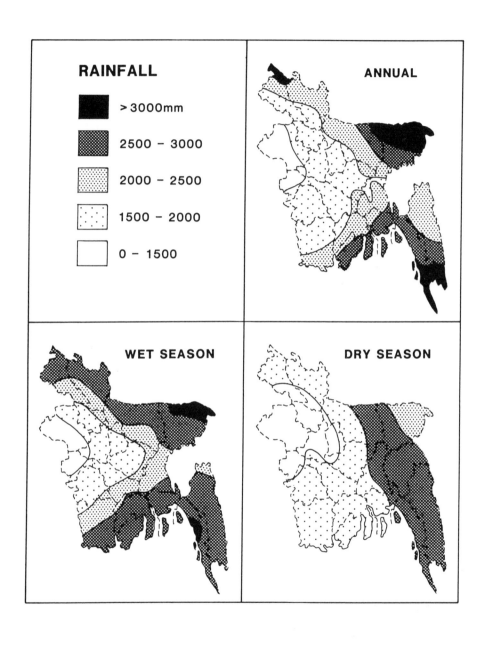

Figure 2.3   Annual and seasonal distribution of rainfall in Bangladesh

Bangladesh. It is the variability of seasonal rainfall that is crucial for the sowing and harvesting of crops on which the food supply depends. For example, the rainfall in the months of May and July is crucial for the sowing of *Aus* and *Aman* crops. The amount of rain in these months affects the size of the crops sown and harvested. The rainfall in these two months is subject to quite large fluctuations as one can see from the rainfall data presented in Table 2.7 for the selected stations. Sometimes the monsoon may end too soon and rain may not be enough for the rice crop in the last month of the monsoon season, Johnson (1975) compared average October rainfall with the October rain in 1935, an exceptional year, to show that even in October the rainfall was not enough for the rice crop over most of the country.

Table 2.7
Rainfall variability

	January	May	July	Annual
DHAKA				
C.V.	134.0	43.5	45.2	14.3
Mean rainfall in inches	0.1	14.6	15.1	86.7
SD	0.2	6.3	6.2	12.4
SYLHET				
CV	146.0	37.8	43.9	22.6
Mean rainfall in inches	0.2	20.2	30.2	159.4
SD	0.3	7.6	13.3	36.0
JESSORE				
CV	156.0	47.5	32.9	22.5
Mean rainfall in inches	0.5	7.6	11.6	67.5
SD	0.8	3.6	3.8	15.2

CV = Coefficient of variability
SD = Standard deviation
Source: Calculated by the author from BBS data

The variability is the highest in the dry winter season, as one would expect. Further, it is higher in the western region which is relatively dry. In January, which is the main sowing time for HYV *Boro* rice, the variability of rainfall is the highest. But because much of the *Boro* rice is irrigated, high variability does not do much damage to the *Boro* rice crop.

Natural hazards

The size of food producing land in Bangladesh in relation to its population is indeed small. Its capacity for food production is further marred by frequent destruction of food crops and animals by natural hazards. Therefore, it appears relevant to discuss them briefly in this chapter.

The location of Bangladesh at the head of the Bay of Bengal combined with its dense population makes it particularly vulnerable to natural hazards. The country is hit almost every year by floods and cyclones. On an average, 3 to 4 tropical cyclones hit the country each year, but some of them may not be too severe; nevertheless, they cause much damage. Floods, cyclones, and infrequent droughts are the most disturbing aspects of Bangladesh climate from the human point of view. They are recurrent features that cause large scale damage to crops, livestock, human life, and non agricultural property.

Floods

An estimated 32,000 sq. miles of the land area in Bangladesh is flood prone, which is more than half the area of the country. About one million acres of land remains under water for periods varying from three to five months every year, with the depth of water varying from a few inches to a few feet.

Depth and frequency of seasonal floods vary considerably across the delta. In the Meghna Esturine Floodplains, Ganges Tidal Floodplains and High Ganges River Floodplains, flooding is generally shallow (Brammer 1993). These three physiographic divisions comprise all the coastal districts, except Chittagong. In this region, the rivers are in their old age and therefore sluggish in their flow. They drop much of the silt and are engaged in land building processes rather than erosion (Spate and Learmonth 1967). In the rest of the country, flooding is moderate to deep during the peak flooding season.

Brammer (1990) has classified floods in Bangladesh into three categories: flash, river, and rain water floods. Flash floods are caused by exceptionally heavy rains in the Himalayan ranges, Khasi and Mizo Hills, which run along the northwestern, northern and eastern borders of Bangladesh. Continuous heavy rain over long periods, during the monsoon season, in the catchment area of the mighty rivers, and heavy rush of water from the hills in the north and east, submerge large areas because river channels are shallow. As most of the major rivers in Bangladesh are exceedingly broad and are being continually filled with alluvium, the rush of water from the north and east is not contained in the streams but overflows and floods large areas. Such floods rise and fall rapidly. Although this is an annual feature, in some years much larger areas are flooded and crop damage is sometimes extensive. The damage to crops is not due to submergence of crops but due to rapidly flowing water, which may uproot plants.

River floods result from melting of snow and heavy rain over extended periods in the Himalayas, the Assam hills and the Tripura hills. Such floods cover much larger areas and bring more water and last considerably longer than flash floods. They cause more damage when they occur early. They uproot crops, cover them with thick alluvial deposits, and erode river banks.

The rain water floods are caused by heavy rain within the country. Heavy pre-monsoon rain, monsoon rain, and overflow from rivers combine to submerge large areas, at some locations to abnormal depths.

The worst floods in the history of the region (including the period under Pakistan and British occupation) occurred in the 1988 summer monsoon season, when 3/4 of the land surface of the nation was submerged under water. Many authorities admitted that it was the most devastating in the living memory . Even the residence of the President was under knee-deep water, and many streets in Dhaka were transformed into canals. An estimated 30 million people were rendered homeless, and more than 3,000 died of drowning, disease, and snake bites (snakes also sought refuge on the same bits of dry land where the homeless population was congregating) during the first week of the floods (*Time* 1988). About half of those left homeless were already facing starvation as many areas were cut off and were unreachable. Many more were believed to die in the next few months due to starvation and water-related diseases.

The crop damage in the 1988 floods was extensive, as was the damage to property. Heavy damage to monsoon crops was done, particularly in the vicinity of Brahamputra and Ganges rives. A large tract in central Bangladesh was also seriously affected. The yield per acre of *Aman* rice crop dropped by more than half a ton per hectare. Consequently, about half the country's population depended on food aid for four to five months after the floods. Montgomery (1985), found that rice production was usually higher in years with high floods, despite substantial loss in some areas. It appears that loss in one area is more than compensated for by increased production in another area. It may be due to higher rainfall in the areas outside the flood damage areas. Also, extra moisture and new silt benefit rabi crops. But this was not true for the 1988 floods because they were extraordinary. The *Aman* production dropped by about 7 percent on the previous year. It did not recover even in 1989. In 1988, *Aman* production was 17 percent below the 1987 level, but *Boro* production was 18 percent above that of 1987. However, the production of *Boro* is only half that of *Aman*, therefore even an in *Boro* did not make up the loss in total rice production.

The 1988 floods followed the inundation of 1987, which was also very serious. Hence, many repairs after the 1987 flood damage were shattered again in 1988 even before they were completely restored. The floods in Bangladesh are not only increasing in fury but also in frequency. The main cause for this is reported to be massive deforestation in India, Nepal, and Bhutan in the catchment areas of the rivers that flow into Bangladesh. Without the vegetation cover the soil has lost its moisture holding capacity. Heavy monsoon rain, therefore, results in savage run off, Which is increasing every year (Curry 1984). The runoff brings large loads of sediments which are dropped on the river beds in Bangladesh due to greatly reduced gradient. These deposits annually raise the river beds and make the surrounding areas more vulnerable to floods. But Ives and Masserli (1989) have strongly refuted this theory. They argue that deforestation in the Himalayas has been going on for several centuries and that high run-off and erosion rates may be attributed to natural processes. There is no evidence that the frequency of floods in Bangladesh has increased or decreased, but the area affected seems to be increasing. There is also no evidence of rising sea levels due to the green-house effects, which will aggravate flooding in Bangladesh by raising river levels.

Large areas become impassable during the annual floods and suffer acute food shortages. During the years of excessive rains, the damage to rice crops from floods may be as high as ten percent, which is more than the normal rice deficit of the country. In 1973-74, an exceptionally bad year for floods, more than a fifth of the rice crop was damaged from floods, causing widespread suffering. The regional pattern of crop damage is quite conspicuous. Sylhet, Kishoreganj, and Faridpur often record the maximum damage from floods, and coastal districts from cyclones and tidal waves.

The Bangladesh Government, with the financial and technical assistance of several developed nations and international agencies, is seriously planning to undertake a flood control program. The Flood Action Plan will include construction of embankments along the full length of all major rivers to carry surplus water during the monsoon period safely to the Bay of Bengal. It will also include embankments around major cities along the rivers. The embankments will be as close as possible to the river to minimize the land area taken by embankments. Along with the construction of embankments the flood plains of the country will be divided into compartments. Each compartment will be treated as a planning unit for food production and integrated rural development. The construction of embankments will start in the upper courses of the rivers and proceed downstream in stages. After the construction of embankments upstream, the flow of water in the downstream channels will increase considerably. Hence, the downstream channels will get time to get adjusted to the increased floods. The increased flow will probably flush some silt from the bottom of the downstream channels into the ocean and thereby deepen the channels. Deeper water in the channels is expected to increase the fish population. It will also be used for controlled flooding during the monsoon season through a series of drains. Some surplus water will be stored for irrigation during the dry winter season.

Some researchers have suggested upstream storage of surplus water during the rainy season in a series of reservoirs and use of this water in the dry season for irrigation. Although this scheme may sound less complex, it is not without problems. Rapid siltation of the reservoirs will be a serious problem, besides other environmental, economic, and social problems. Where will the dams and reservoirs be located? Which villages will have to go? Who will benefit most from the scheme? How safe will it be to locate huge dams in a geologically unstable area? These are some of the important questions that must be seriously considered before launching the scheme.

Some have suggested the dredging of the river channels, which have become

38

very shallow due to silting. Along with dredging, a massive reforestation program on the southern slopes of the Himalayas in Nepal, Bhutan, and India will reduce siltation. But such an ambitious program will require the cooperation of all four countries, for which the present political atmosphere does not appear very encouraging.

Droughts

In a region where annual average rainfall is in excess of 2,500 mm, it is rather hard to imagine droughts as serious natural hazards. Although droughts are relatively infrequent in Bangladesh, they do cause widespread crop failures and usher in severe famines. Droughts are, in fact, a characteristic feature of monsoon climates, and are related to the uncertainty of monsoon rains. In spite of heavy rainfall characteristics of the Bangladesh climate, the year to year variations in the amount are quite significant. The failure of monsoons is well known to the inhabitants of South Asia, but in Bangladesh it is not so frequent.

Of the three types of droughts, i.e., meteorological, hydrological, and agricultural, only agricultural drought is important in the context of Bangladesh. Agricultural drought results when the monsoon rain is not enough or does not come at the right time for the established cropping pattern. Because Bangladesh is generally a wet region, different varieties of rice and jute — water loving crops — dominate the cropping pattern. However, when the monsoon fails the rainfall may be less than the requirement for rice, jute, and sugar cane, which grow during the summer monsoon period. When the monsoon fails, conditions become very dry in winter, and make it difficult for even less moisture-demanding crops to grow. Hence, failure to the monsoon not only affects summer crops but also winter crops (Figure 2.4). Rice being the most widespread crop, the damage to rice crops is large, and often the production drops by 20 percent. As revealed in figure 2.4, the impact of drought is clearly uneven across regions. It may be noted that the adverse impact of drought is minimal on *Aman* rice , which is grown during the summer monsoon months. This implies that even reduced rainfall is often enough for the crops grown during the rainy season. The failure of the summer monsoon is more felt during the dry winter season. It is interesting to note that the impact of drought on low lying areas such as those in Sylhet, Mymensingh, and coastal districts, for the summer crops, appears to be positive, indicating that in the low areas excess moisture during the summer monsoon is the major problem for crop production. Therefore, a drop in moisture supply during occasional droughts increases rather than decreases the output of summer crops in such areas (Figure 3c). The maximum damage by drought is done to the winter crops such as *Boro*, because during the drought years there is little soil moisture left in the soil by then, and a low level or absence of water in the streams and ponds reduces the proportion of winter crop areas irrigated.

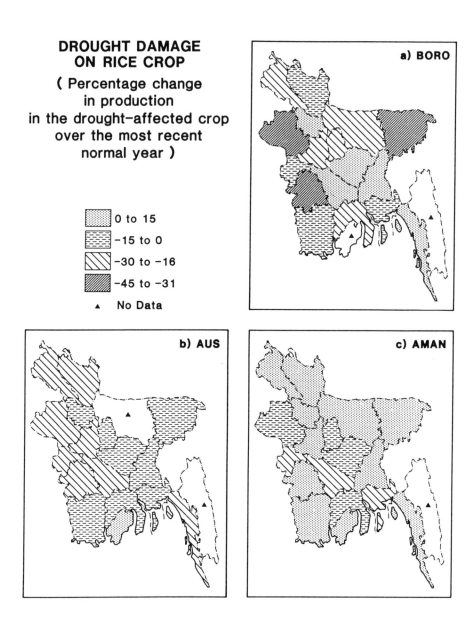

DROUGHT DAMAGE ON RICE CROP

(Percentage change in production in the drought−affected crop over the most recent normal year)

0 to 15
−15 to 0
−30 to −16
−45 to −31
▲ No Data

a) BORO

b) AUS

c) AMAN

Figure 2.4 Regional drought damage on rice crop

A number of weak shallow tropical depressions develop in the Bay of Bengal along the Inter Tropical Convergence Zone due to mixing of air of very different temperatures and humidities. Despite being weak, such depressions are able to produce a lot of convective precipitation. They are responsible for much of the monsoon rain in Bangladesh and India. Sometimes, one of these weak depressions develop into a violent cyclone that may cause much damage to standing crops, livestock, and property.

The pre-monsoon and post-monsoon months are characterized by sometimes severe cyclonic activities. The most cyclone-prone regions of Bangladesh are in the coastal districts of Khulna, Patuakhali, Barisal, and Chittagong, and off-shore islands. These cyclonic storms are caused by a sudden drop in atmospheric pressure well below the normal. Winds associated with cyclones often reach velocities up to 200 miles per hour, and generate sea waves as high as 50 feet. When a wall of water of this size strikes land with massive force the damage done to life and property can be easily imagined. The damage done by tropical cyclones is related to three main causes: strong winds, river flooding from sudden heavy rains, and coastal flooding from storm surges. So the damage to life and property is not so much from winds, but from the effects of flooding. The world distribution of storms on a map clearly shows an unusual concentration in the Bay of Bengal (Anthes 1981). The frequency of major cyclones is quite high, averaging about two per year. During the 11 year period ending in December 1970, out of 19 major cyclone disasters in the world, 5 occurred in Bangladesh. More recently, between 1971 and 1992, Bangladesh was hit by 21 severe cyclones. The cyclone of November 1970, that culminated in the death of 300,000 people and crop damage of millions of dollars. The fearful cyclone wiped out over half the population in some areas of the coastal belt of Patuakhali and Noakhali districts. It destroyed 65 percent of the coastal fishing capacity, seriously depleting protein supply (Whitlow 1980). In April 1991, Bangladesh was hit by the strongest cyclone of this century, but the loss of life was not as great as in the 1970 cyclone because of greater preparedness. Bangladesh now has a complex ten-level cyclone warning system, and about 300 multistoried shelters in the low lying coastal districts have been built. Officials think that about 3,000 shelters are needed to provide adequate protection to the population in the coastal districts.

Floods and cyclones are the two key elements affecting wide fluctuations in agricultural output. The damage to crops is large because floods and cyclones usually hit the nation during the planting or harvesting of crops. Hence, the incidence of material damage by natural hazards in Bangladesh is perhaps higher than in any other country of Asia, if not in the world. The damage by natural hazards could well be a major cause of poverty in Bangladesh, as more than 75 percent of its population depends directly on agricultural activities.

Agricultural labour and draft animals

In an intensive food production system carried out on small holdings, labour is the most important input. Fortunately, this is the only resource required for food production for which there is no scarcity in Bangladesh.

In the developed nations, the agricultural labour force has been consistently declining because it is being increasingly replaced by machinery. As a consequence, growing number of consumers in these countries are becoming increasingly dependent for food on a shrinking labour force in agriculture. In contrast, in Bangladesh, an increasing quantity of food is being supplied by an increasing labour force.

The labour force in Bangladesh is composed of all able-bodied individuals above 10 years of age. The labour force data, particularly for the agricultural labour force in Bangladesh, are rather confusing. The labour force data are collected under population censuses, agricultural censuses, and labour force surveys. The figures published by the relevant three organizations are not commensurate. They differ probably because of differences in definitions and coverage. Within each organization too the definitions and coverage have changed over time. Hence, an accurate analysis of the growth of the labour force is not possible. The BBS has published civilian force data for 1974, 1981, 1983-84, 1984-85, 1985-86, 1989, and 1991 that have been adjusted for under-count, over-count, and unemployed persons, but not for changes in definitions. There was a big jump in the female labour force in 1989 due to inclusion of several additional activities, mainly carried out by women, as agricultural labour (Table 2.8).

In 1974, about 14 million persons were employed in agriculture. If the data provided in Table 2.7 are reasonably correct, they indicate that the growth in the size of the male agricultural labour force has been quite spectacular. Between 1974 and 1991, it increased by 28.6 percent or at the annual rate of 1.7 percent. The growth in the female labour force in 1989 was exceptional due to changes in definitions. Because of changes in the definitions, the female participation in the agricultural labour force is now 43 percent. Until 1989, a lot of activities that are carried out by women such as care of animals and poultry, boiling paddy, and food processing and preservation were not counted as agricultural labour. The new data show that women are very actively involved in agricultural activities.

Over time, the increasing labour force has been continually channelled into agriculture. As a result, agriculture has become so labour intensive that despite an abundant supply of labour, there is some shortage of labour in the peak season. According to one estimate, labour demand reaches a maximum of 310 labour days per acre in the month of May (Iqbal 1978). It means that in the rice growing areas in May the labour requirement reaches 10 workers per acre per day. This clearly indicates that labour is the most important input in the food production systems of Bangladesh.

No data are published on the quality of the agricultural labour force, i.e., their educational training levels. But a low level of literacy (less than 25 percent) one would expect the quality to be very low. Until recently, not much investment was made in lifting the educational and training levels in the rural areas. Even after independence, the allocation of funds to different sectors indicates no significant increase for education and training through successive plans. The investment in 'human capital' has not been very significant. Schultz's hypothesis in the context of Bangladesh suggests that there is urgent need for increasing public investment in education and training of the labour force (Schultz 1964). This is required to improve the quality of the labour force, which will eventually increase productivity of labour.

Table 2.8
Agricultural labour force
(Figures in millions)

Years	Males	Females
1974	13.6	0.46
1981	15.2	0.93
1983-84	16.1	1.50
1984-85	16.1	1.60
1985-86	16.8	1.90
1989	18.7	13.90
1990	17.5	12.85

Source: Compiled from the data in the Statistical Yearbooks of Bangladesh, various issues
Note: The data for 1981 were estimated from civilian rural labour force data, because the employment data in that year were not classified in the same major employment categories as in other years

Rapidly increasing labour input in constant land leads towards a tendency to diminishing returns. This is believed to be happening in several developing countries where it is depressing the output per unit of labour (Myrdal 1977). Amazingly enough, in Bangladesh, this does not seem to be happening. During the 1970s and 1980s labour productivity increased at the rate of 5.5 percent per year; in fact it increased faster than land productivity (Dayal 1990). The trend of labour productivity over time will be discussed in more detail later in Chapter 5.

The 1983-84 Agricultural Census indicated that at that time 63 percent of the non-farm households were agricultural labour households. Some farm households were also classified as agricultural labour households, because their main source of income was from agricultural labour. This is quite common in Bangladesh. Many farm households have very little land, and therefore besides cultivating their own land they also have to work as agricultural labourers to earn enough to support the

43

household. About 31 percent of the farm household happen to be in this category.

The purely agricultural labour households, who do not have any land of their own to cultivate, augment their incomes by going into a number of subsidiary economic activities such as raising a few cattle, sheep or goats, and poultry. But the most popular among these is poultry keeping, which has been promoted by the government and non-government organizations alike as part of their hunger and poverty eradication programs. Poultry farming needs little training and capital, and is largely carried out by women, who are otherwise not part of the labour force. Interestingly enough, a very small proportion of the agricultural labour households is engaged in cottage industries. The pattern of subsidiary economic activities for agricultural labour households who have no land and those who have some land to cultivate is practically the same.

The regional distribution of agricultural labour households is quite distinctive. For some reason, they are concentrated in all the border districts, all along the northern and western borders. In this contiguous region, the percentage of agricultural labour households is well above the national average.

In Bangladesh, as in most other Asian countries, all agricultural operations are carried out by using human and animal power. Although there is practically no land that can be spared for growing fodder crops, Bangladesh has a large cattle population that is largely raised on crop residues (Jansen 1986). Husk, bran, straw, leaves, stalks, and stones of fruit crops such as mango and jack fruit are fed to livestock. The milk yields of bovine animals are very low. However, the usefulness of cattle and buffaloes should not be judged only in terms of milk yields. They contribute to the prosperity of peasants in more important ways than providing milk only. They are the main source of draft power and also supply milk, meat, dung for manure, hides, and bones. Bangladesh had 21 million cattle and 400,000 buffaloes at the time of 1984-83 agricultural census. Of the total, about 17 million were adults (more than 3 years old). About 70 percent of the adult cattle and buffaloes are defined as working cattle, and 90 percent of these are used in a variety of agricultural operations. The rest provide draft power for several other activities such as transport, and crushing oil seeds and sugarcane. Thus, cattle and buffaloes should be considered an important part of agricultural capital.

Because of their importance as draft animals, 95 percent of the bovine animals are possessed by farm households. The density of bovine animals on cultivated land is fairly uniform throughout Bangladesh, with the notable exception of Chittagong, where it is one and a half times the national average. In all the other districts, the density of bovine animals on cultivated land deviates only slightly above and below the national average. The density of bovine animals on small farms is twice as high as on the large farms. This is because each small farmer tries to be independent in the supply of draft power.

Normally a good pair of bullocks can plough half an acre in a day, and is sufficient for a holding of 10 to 15 acres. But after the first few monsoon rains, ploughing of the field must be completed as quickly as possible. Therefore, during the peak season there is often a shortage of draft animals, making it impossible for small farmers to borrow or hire draft animals. Hence, it is necessary for each farmer to keep a pair of draft animals irrespective of the size of their holding.

Besides bovine animals, there were about 14 million sheep and goats in Bangladesh. About 86 percent of sheep and goats are possessed by farm households, more than half of them by small farm households. Sheep and goats are an important source of supplementary income. They multiply fast, provide some milk, and are easy to sell for meat in the market. They are not expensive to raise because they can survive on stubble, leaves and stalks of banana trees, and some crop residue. They can also graze on thorny bushes. All that is required is some labour for tending the animals. In small farm households, there is always some surplus labour, because there is not enough work on the small holdings.

Keeping poultry is a growing supplementary activity in Bangladesh. Between the 1977 and 1983-84 agricultural censuses, the poultry birds in the country increased by 37 percent. Poultry raising again is an ideal supplementary activity for small farm households, because it is inexpensive and very space efficient. Therefore, small farm households displayed the greatest increase of 88 percent between the two censuses. A very high percentage of farm households (85) possessed poultry. The remaining 15 percent were owned by the non-farm households. Poultry keeping is very helpful activity, particularly for the small farmers, because it provides some cash income throughout the year. It is particularly helpful during the periods before the harvests, when small farms face acute shortages of food.

Resource endowment and the future

Despite decreasing size of land resources in Bangladesh, their food producing capacity has been consistently increasing. The major contributors to the increased food producing capacity of land resources are higher multiple cropping and average yields, which are due to greater use of HYRV seeds, fertilizers, and irrigation. The Flood Action Plan which is now under way will further augment the food production capacity of land resources. It will not only reduce crop damage but also increase crop yields for summer crops from controlled flooding and in winter from increased irrigation. Increased volume of water in the deeper river channels and some reservoirs will make winter irrigation expansion more feasible and less expensive. The irrigation expansion will also reduce the effect of droughts on food production.

Although cyclones will continue to damage standing food crops and reduce food supply whenever they hit the country, greater preparedness might help reduce the loss of livestock and property. Thus without being too optimistic, one may suggest that the future of food supply appears promising.

Summary

Although the farm land in Bangladesh is very fertile, there is an acute shortage of it. Hence, the resource base for food production is limited. During the period under review, the area of cultivated land remained virtually unchanged, while the population increased by 44 percent. Therefore the level of landlessness among the rural population is high and increasing. The net cropped area per head of the agricultural population declined considerably during the period. This has led to more frequent use of the existing cropland, which may threaten land productivity.

The ownership of land is heavily concentrated in a few hands. About 10 percent of the large landowners own 50 percent of the farm land. Consequently, 70 percent of the agricultural holdings are less than 2.5 acres and often highly fragmented.

Bangladesh has a warm humid sub-tropical climate with a wet summer and dry winter. Winters are so dry that only 20 percent of the net cropped area is cultivated during the winter. A dominant feature of the climate is a high frequency of natural hazards such as floods, cyclones, and droughts.

3 Agricultural landscape

Ten major crops, cultivated over a large number of small holdings, dominate the agricultural landscape in Bangladesh. With the exception of jute they are all food crops (Table 3.1). They occupy 90 percent of the total cropped area (TCA) in the country and about 80 percent or more in each district, except Chittagong HT. Hence, the ten selected crops adequately represent the cropping pattern in Bangladesh and were considered suitable for analysing crop pattern change. In this chapter, the dynamics of crop pattern, ranking crops, and crop regions will be discussed.

Table 3.1

Cropping pattern: area under ten major crops as a percentage of total cropped area for 1971-74 and 1989-92

(Four year averages)

Crop	1971-74	1989-92
Aman	44.4	43.8
Boro	06.9	11.6
Aus	24.9	21.6
Wheat	01.0	04.5
Masur	00.6	00.5
Moong	00.2	00.1
Kheseri	00.7	00.6
Gram	00.5	00.4
Mashkali	00.4	00.2
Jute	06.6	06.5

Source: calculated by the author from BBS data

The term cropping pattern refers to the way crops share the cropland during an agricultural year. The cropping pattern in any region is determined by a set of socio-economic and physical factors. In Bangladesh, the cropping pattern is dependent on eight major factors, i.e., climate, topography, soils, local customs and traditions, irrigation development, costs and availability of inputs, demand and utility of crops, and marketing facilities (BBS 1986). For example, physical environments in Bangladesh are not ideal for some crops that thrive better in drier climates. Nevertheless, crops like wheat, bajra, and gram, which do better in relatively drier conditions, are successfully cultivated in Bangladesh in winter, because winters are quite dry. The socio-economic environment in Bangladesh, on the other hand, would not justify some agricultural activities. For example, scarcity of land and capital would not permit cattle raising or extensive mechanized crop farming. The existing pattern is heavily dependent on demand for food. The rapid growth of population, particularly during the last two decades, created enormous demand for food. Therefore, the cropping pattern in Bangladesh has become more dominated by food crops, which occupy 92 percent of the total cropped area. Foodgrains alone, which include cereals and pulses, account for 82 percent of the cropped area. Despite the relative weakness of the cash crops in the cropping pattern, they are desperately needed for earning foreign exchange in an otherwise resource poor country. For example, jute is a major source of foreign exchange earnings, but it occupies only 5 percent of the cropped area.

Although the size and distribution of the cultivated area changed little in Bangladesh over time, some very substantial changes have occurred in the cropping pattern. In an effort to maximize agricultural output, particularly food, for an increasing population, the available cultivated land is being used quite differently in the 1990s from how it was in the 1970s. The major change is an increase in the area sown to foodgrains. Despite these changes the cropping pattern continues to be dominated by rice. Wheat, a recently introduced crop, has now become the second ranking cereal crop. The area under both these important food crops increased during the period by 5 percent and 300 percent respectively. As there has been little change in the net cultivated area, the increase in the area under rice and wheat is presumably at the expense of decline in fallow or an increase in multiple cropping.

Food crops

Rice

Rice is intensively cultivated wherever possible and completely dominates the agricultural landscape. It now occupies 92.34 percent of the total cereals area, and 80 percent off the total cropped area, and forms 86 percent of the cereal production. In the 1983-84 agricultural census, it was found that all rural households were involved in some rice cultivation. Bangladesh occupies fourth place in rice production in the world after India, China, and Japan. China and India are both much bigger producers of rice, producing more than twice as much as Bangladesh.

The conditions for rice cultivation are ideal in Bangladesh. In fact, it is believed to be one of the areas where rice was originally domesticated. The botanical variety grown in Bangladesh is *oryza savita*. Until the release of High Yielding Rice Varieties (HYRVs), there were three main varieties of rice in Bangladesh: *Aman*, *Boro*, and *Aus*. Each of these has several sub-varieties, determined by the fineness and length of the grain. Fine long grain varieties fetch higher prices in the market because they are preferred by the urban consumers. The introduction of High Yielding Varieties (HYVs) has greatly increased the varieties which are now cultivated in Bangladesh. Now there are traditional and HYVs of each of the three main rice crops. In the following discussion, each main crop includes both varieties.

Among the varieties of rice cultivated, *Aman* is undoubtedly by far the most important. It is cultivated during the monsoon season and largely depends on rainfall. Based on the method of cultivation, three types of *Aman* rice are identified- transplant *Aman*, broadcast *Aman*, and HYV *Aman*. Transplanted *Aman* occupies nearly half the area under rice in the country and also accounts for about half the rice supply .

The broadcast *Aman* is the traditional rice variety in Bangladesh and is next in importance. It is cultivated in low lying areas that are deeply flooded during the monsoon season. Hence, it is also known as deep water rice or floating rice. Broadcast *Aman* is sown before the monsoons in March and April and harvested after the monsoons in November. Some varieties of broadcast rice are ready for harvesting by September, when the flood water is still quite deep in the fields, and are harvested by boats. It can grow with rising water and can often reach a height of more than 15 feet. Although its yield per acre is relatively low, it contributes a significant amount to the rice supply of Bangladesh. An important feature of broadcast rice is that it is grown in very low lying areas which would otherwise remain unused for crop production during the monsoon season. The HYV *Aman* has not yet become very popular because it requires controlled water conditions for fertilizer application to be more effective. Also, in deeply submerged areas the application of fertilizers and manure is not very effective as they cannot be retained in the specified fields. Sometimes it may even work against the crop if washed down in the nearby weed infested areas that often invade floating rice. Therefore, the percentage of area under HYV *Aman* is much smaller than under other varieties. The distribution of *Aman* in Bangladesh is so widespread that there is hardly any spatial concentration. Nevertheless, the southeastern districts appear to have a somewhat higher density than other parts of Bangladesh.

The area under *Aman* rice has increased little in recent years relative to other rice crops. The large area already under *Aman* rice and its heavy dependence on monsoon rains probably limit the scope for expansion. The *Aman* cultivation has already stretched to its practical limits, and therefore its acreage is unlikely to expand any further. Also, jute, the major cash crop of Bangladesh, also competes for a share of the cropland with *Aman* during the monsoon season.

The *Boro* rice crop, often called winter rice, is now second in importance both in terms of area and production. This is largely due to the rapid spread of HYV *Boro* in the 1980s. In the 1970s, *Aus* contributed more to area and production than *Boro*, but not any more. Because it is grown in winter, which is the dry season, it depends on irrigation. This is the only rice crop in Bangladesh for which water control and use of fertilizers are most effective, therefore, it has benefited most from the HYVs. Because of controlled water supply and application of fertilizers *Boro* rice gives much heavier average yield than *Aus* or *Aman*. It yields twice that of *Aus* and one and a half times that of *Aman* per acre. Among the rice crops, therefore, acreage under *Boro* has recorded the most impressive increase in recent years. Although wheat and *Boro* rice are cultivated in the same season they do not compete against each other for land because they occupy different areas. *Boro* requires more water than wheat therefore it is cultivated in the low lying areas or in the areas where irrigation is available. Greater stability and development of small irrigation are important factors that have contributed to the expansion of *Boro* rice in Bangladesh. *Boro* is sown in December and harvested in April. Because it is harvested in spring it is called by some the spring rice crop. *Boro* stays in the fields during the winter season therefore it is least damaged by natural hazards. Geographical concentration of *Boro* is clearly in the northeast, mainly in the Sylhet Basin. The monsoon water collects in this depression but its level is too high for other rice crops during the monsoon season. After the monsoon season the depth of water begins to recede and in winters the depth is ideal for *Boro* rice.

Aus is third in importance, both in terms of area and production. It is also sown broadcast in low lying areas before the real onset of monsoons, and is locally known as *Bhadoi* rice. It is harvested in August and September by boats, because the flood water in the fields is still very high for normal harvesting. *Aus* contributes about a quarter of the total rice supply in Bangladesh. The growing popularity of *Boro* has not adversely affected the area under *Aus* because the two crops are cultivated in different seasons. *Aus* has, however, some concentration in the eastern districts. The acreage under *Aus* has declined, perhaps as a result of the expansion of the two other rice crops. There is some overlap in the sowing seasons of *Aus* and *Aman*, and some overlap in the sowing of *Aus* and the harvesting of *Boro*. Therefore, expansion of *Aman* and *Boro* is likely to result in a shrinkage in the area under *Aus*.

Despite the fact that every inch of the arable land suitable for rice cultivation is used for it, its area over time has continued to increase. During the two decades ending in 1992, the area under rice crop increased by 12 percent but the production increased by 35 percent. Obviously this happened through significant increases in productivity. The average yield per acre of all rice varieties during the same period increased by 29 percent, largely due to high yielding variety seeds and associated increases in the use of irrigation and fertilizers. The increase in rice production was much more impressive in the central, west-central, and coastal districts of Bangladesh, which are relatively less populated. The increase in the eastern and southeastern districts has been below average. This is perhaps an indication that intensity of cultivation has almost reached saturation point and any further increase in rural population will only worsen the food situation. In Sylhet, rice production declined during the period, but this was more than compensated for by an increase in wheat production.

Wheat

Wheat is a relatively new crop in Bangladesh but it has recorded the most impressive increase in both area and production during the last 20 years (Table 3.2).

Table 3.2
Wheat in Bangladesh

	1972-74	1980-82	1990-91
Area (000 ha)	301	1390	1450
Yield Kg/ha	344	729	714
Production (000 tons)	103	1013	1035

Source: Calculated by the author from BBS data

Wheat began to be promoted in Bangladesh in the 1960s. The idea for wheat production emerged when Bangladesh began to import large quantities of wheat to wipe off the persisting food deficit. There was an acute shortage of rice in 1973, which encouraged the government to promote wheat more enthusiastically. They established hundreds of demonstration farms. Although people have a strong preference for rice, importing rice is more expensive as none of the major exporters of foodgrains has a large surplus of rice available for export. This situation left Bangladesh with no choice but to import wheat from wherever available. Large imports of wheat must have initiated some change in the food habits of the people. Nowadays, western style loaves of bread, biscuits, and Indian style bread all made from wheat flour are commonly used by people in most households at least for breakfast.

Wheat area during the period increased by more than 382 percent. The introduction and rapid expansion of wheat in Bangladesh is a particularly welcome change in many ways. Some unirrigated land that remained idle during dry winters, because of inadequate soil moisture for rice, is now profitably used for wheat production. Its introduction has increased the level of multiple cropping and contributed significantly to an overall increase in the area under foodgrains. In some districts, the area under wheat cultivation increased more than 600 times during the period. Hence, its contribution to increasing food supply in Bangladesh cannot be exaggerated. A similar pattern of change is also discernible from the production figures, but the change in production is much greater than the increases in area.

The yield per acre of most crops increased during the last two decades in Bangladesh, but the increase was most spectacular for wheat. The yield per acre of wheat more than doubled during the period under consideration. This rather unusual increase in the yield per acre of wheat is because it is a new crop in Bangladesh,

51

introduced only in the 1960s. The initial response of farmers to wheat promotion campaigns was cold. But rapid population growth and some improvement in incomes increased the demand for food and made the food deficit situation worse. Thus, the worsening food deficit and some change in food habits generated some interest in wheat cultivation. Initially most farmers must have been quite ignorant about the cultivation techniques of wheat. But the subsequent success of wheat, as a new food crop in Bangladesh, must have generated greater interest and care in its cultivation, leading to diversion of more inputs and efforts into its cultivation. Hence, yield per acre increased more rapidly. Further, wheat benefited more from the HYV program throughout south Asia. The total area under wheat increased much more than under rice. This is of course understandable. Rice has been the main crop in Bangladesh since time immemorial, therefore, it has already been stretched as far as practical. The ecological requirements of rice are much more demanding. In Bangladesh, water supply is the major constraint for rice cultivation. In the winter season, conditions do not permit rice cultivation, except in the irrigated or low lying areas where soil moisture is sufficient. Therefore, wheat, which requires little moisture, has now proved an ideal winter crop. Yet another reason for its rapid expansion is its greater stability. The growing period of wheat, like that of *Boro* rice, is not much affected by natural disasters. This makes it a safer crop for investment in new inputs and a more reliable source of food supply. Wheat cultivation is distinctly concentrated in the west-central districts of Bangladesh, notably Faridpur, Kushtia, Pabna, and Rajshahi. There is virtually no cultivation of wheat in the coastal districts, which are too wet for the crop even in winter.

In wheat was found an excellent solution for reducing the food deficit in the country. With the help of some development aid, the government of Bangladesh sent some agricultural scientists to Mexico for training in HYV wheat cultivation. On their return, they demonstrated that they could produce 800 to 1200 kg/ac of wheat without irrigation during the dry winter season on land that otherwise remained unused due to insufficient soil moisture for rice. On irrigated land, up to 2,000 kg of wheat could be produced on one acre of land. It can be cultivated in several areas without irrigation because it requires much loss water, only 300-450 ml compared with 800-1600 ml for rice (Hanson and Norman 1982). The government encouraged wheat cultivation by providing a guarantied price to wheat producers, which was kept above the world market price. The government employed a mixed strategy for wheat promotion. It was based on a national campaign for wheat promotion, demonstration farms across the country, maintaining adequate supply of seeds and a good system of distribution, creation and training of extension staff, and agronomic research. This strategy proved very successful and led to rapid expansion of wheat. In its expansion program, Bangladesh benefited much from Indian experience. The main wheat variety now cultivated is *sonalika* developed in India. But Bangladesh has also developed two new varieties — *balaka* and *dod* — to suit local conditions.

One notable change in the cropping pattern in Bangladesh agriculture appears to be a gradual decline in the acreage of low market value coarse grain crops, i.e., maize, jowar, bajra, and barley (Table 3.1). The maximum percentage decline is for barley, because it grows during the same season as wheat and *Boro* rice, and it has to compete for a share of the cropland with these two rapidly expanding crops. The reason for the decline of coarse grains appears to be greater profitability in rice and wheat caused by the expansion of minor irrigation projects and HYV seeds. This is definitely good news for the cultivators, as it augments their incomes. But it is bad news for the poor, who are the main consumers of coarse grains, as the shortage of coarse grains has increased their prices. Although the change towards larger a area under rice and wheat has increased their supply, it has not caused any relative decline in their prices. Therefore, it is very likely that the change has worsened the food intake of the very poor in the rural areas, at least in the short run.

Pulses

Pulses are very important in the average diet of the people in Bangladesh. Although Bangladesh is a Muslim country and the majority of the population is non-vegetarian, most people cannot afford meat regularly because of very low incomes. Therefore, pulses are the main source of protein for them. Pulses, being leguminous crops, are an important source of supplying nitrogen to the soils. Hence, pulses are important in affecting not only the nutritional status of the people but also agricultural productivity. It is, therefore, disturbing to note that the area under pulses has been consistently declining over the last two decades. The index number for the acreage for pulses has declined from 100 in 1972-73 to 78 in 1992. But the data for pulses prior to 1983-84 are not comparable to data after that year. In the agricultural census 1983-84, it was found that the acreage for pulses was under-reported, hence, production figures were also incorrect. Therefore, changes in the areal strength of pulses in the cropping pattern can only be assessed from the agricultural census years 1983-84 (Table 3.3).

Table 3.3
Area and production of pulses
(3 year averages)

	1983-86	1989-92
Area (000 acres)	1250	1363
Production (000 metric tons)	350	392

Source: Calculated by the author from BBS data

There are several different types of pulses that are cultivated in Bangladesh, but *Khesari, Masur, Mashkali, Moong*, and gram are the leading types. Together these five accounted for 3.8 percent of the TCA in 1983-84, but dropped to 3.9 percent in

53

1992. The cultivation of pulses is mainly concentrated in the west central districts, where, in terms of area, Faridpur, Jessore, Barisal, Rajshahi, Pabna and Kushtia are the five leading districts in that order. But their ranks have changed over time. In 1992, Faridkot became the leading district in the acreage and production of pulses.

Fruits and vegetables

The physical and human environments in Bangladesh are ideal for the cultivation of vegetables. Soil is fertile and well drained, except in the low lying areas. The temperatures are high enough to permit year round cultivation of a variety of vegetables. Because most vegetables can be harvested within three months of planting, vegetable cultivation permits more intensive use of land than is possible with cereals. This is a big advantage particularly for the small farmers. Further, vegetable farming is much more labour intensive than cereals; therefore it provides more work for the otherwise underemployed labour force.

In terms of area, vegetables and fruits do not appear very important in the cropping pattern because they occupy only small areas. For example, vegetables — including potatoes and sweet potatoes — occupy only 2.7 percent of the TCA. But their importance in the food supply is much greater than is portrayed by the proportion of cropped area they occupy. This is because vegetables yield three to five times more per acre than cereals and pulses. Vegetables are also important because they are a relatively cheap and affordable source of vitamins and minerals in the average diet of the people. The first six major vegetables are potatoes, brinjals, pumpkins, cauliflowers, cabbage, and watergourd in that order. There are also several varieties of beans, gourds, and leafy vegetables which are grown widely.

There is an apparent lack of regional concentration of vegetable farming. In the absence of good roads and fast transport, every district has its own vegetable farming. Nevertheless, there is some concentration in the northwestern and western districts presumably due to availability of more irrigation facilities. There is a marked concentration of brinjal and pumpkin cultivation in Jessore, Bogra, Rangpur, and Rajshahi districts.

Fruits are even less important than vegetables in terms of area occupied, but they too provide a relatively cheap source of several vitamins. Due to lack of a canning and cold storage industry, fruits are quite cheap in season. Fruits occupy only 1.2 percent of the cropped area. The leading fruits are mango, banana, and jackfruit. These three together occupy 70 percent of the total area under fruits. Again some concentration of mango is noticeable in the northwestern districts and of banana in the coastal districts. Jackfruits are grown almost everywhere on small areas. In fact, a few jackfruit trees are grown in the courtyard of almost every dwelling in rural Bangladesh.

Cash crops

In a densely populated country such as Bangladesh, where the land/people ratio is small and declining, it is not difficult to understand the relative unimportance of cash crops in the cropping pattern. Cash crops occupy only 7 percent of the gross cropped area. In the absence of minerals, forests, and manufactures, it is essential to grow some cash crops to earn foreign exchange that is necessary to pay for imports. Jute, sugarcane, and tobacco are the three leading cash crops in Bangladesh.

Jute

Jute is the most important cash crop, occupying approximately 1.50 million acres. Before the partition of the subcontinent, 80 percent of the world's jute was produced in the area now occupied by Bangladesh, but the situation has now changed. India, China, Burma, Thailand, and Brazil have now become important producers of jute. Bangladesh is now the second largest producer of jute after India, producing a little less than a million tonnes annually (Table 3.4).

Table 3.4
Area, yield, and production of jute

	(3 year averages)	
	1972-74	1990-92
Area (000ac)	2205	1447
Yield Kg/ac	838	661
Production (000 Metric tons)	6257	957

Source: Calculated by the author from BBS data

Ideal ecological conditions for jute cultivation are found in the deltas of tropical rivers as it requires deep alluvial soils having ample moisture. Both these conditions are fully met in Bangladesh. It requires a warm and humid environment for a period of about 5 months for successful cultivation. The jute plant probably originated in China from where, it is believed, it must have been brought into India. In Bangladesh, jute is cultivated during the monsoon season. Unlike rice, young plants of jute are somewhat sensitive to waterlogging, therefore, planting is done a few months before heavy the monsoon rains. Hence, before the water level in the fields begin to rise in July and August, jute plants are strong and tall enough to tolerate standing water. The crop is usually sown broadcast. After the plants are about 6 inches tall, thinning is done by hand to reduce the density to about 2,000 plants per acre.

Jute is mainly cultivated for export either as a raw material or in the form of finished jute products. In the 1970s, the situation was desperate because after independence jute was the only foreign exchange earner left in the new country. During the last two decades the area under jute has fluctuated considerably. The two year average for 1972-74 was about 2.2 million acres. In the mid 1970s, it dropped to about 1.6 million acres, but increased again towards the late 1980s to reach the 1970s level. The two year average for 1990-92 was only 1.4 million acres, which was 36 percent below the 1972-74 level. Despite these fluctuations, jute continues to be the most important commercial crop and foreign exchange earner. Jute cultivation in Bangladesh has received some set-back in recent years due to changes in profitability relative to rice. A comparison of net profitability in traditional varieties of rice and jute indicates that jute was a more profitable crop to grow before the introduction of HYVs. Now the position has reversed. In the improved varieties, the costs have increased for both rice and jute, but the value of output per acre has increased much more for rice, making rice a more profitable crop to grow (Islam 1984). Therefore, it is likely that jute acreage in the 1990s may decline. This may also happen due to increasing pressure for achieving self sufficiency in food supply.

Jute is cultivated almost everywhere in Bangladesh except in very low lying tracts such as the Sylhet Basin and coastal districts. Nevertheless, there is some concentration along the Brahamaputra and Padma rivers.

Sugar cane

Sugar cane is the second most important commercial crop in Bangladesh for which suitable ecological conditions are quite widespread in the country (Table 3.5). Sugar cane is crushed to make white sugar in the modern sugar factories and *gur* (unrefined sugar) by traditional methods in villages, both of which are widely consumed by the urban and rural populations. Hence, sugar cane is both an important food crop and a commercial crop. It is the only commercial crop under which the area in recent years has increased despite increasing demand for land for foodgrains.

Sugar cane is concentrated in the relatively higher western districts, namely, Bogra, Rajshahi, Kushtia, and southern half of Dinajpur, districts. Besides these major concentrations, some minor concentrations exist in Dhaka, Mymensingh, and Patuakhali districts.

Tobacco

Tobacco is the third ranking commercial crop. The area under tobacco in recent years has declined. Tobacco cultivation is very labour intensive and requires rich soil for successful cultivation. From both these points of view, Bangladesh is well suited for its cultivation. For this reason, perhaps, the Ganges delta was a major tobacco producing region in British India. Since independence the area under tobacco has recorded some increase. Tobacco cultivation is mainly concentrated in the districts of Rangpur and Kushtia, which account for about 75 percent of the area under the crop.

56

Table 3.5
Area under commercial crops

Crops	Acreage (000ac)	
	1972-74	1990-92
Jute	2205	1447
Sugar cane	331	467
Tobacco	108	93
Cotton	20	NA

Source: Calculated by the author BBS data

Ranking crops

Cropland under all environmental conditions is shared by a variety of crops, but over time some crops become more dominant than others in the cropping pattern. The ranking of crops, on the basis of their relative share of the cropland, is a useful exercise as it provides a primary understanding of the regional dominance of different crops in a given country. Further, a comparison of crop ranks over time in given areas provide a broad picture of the major changes in the cropping pattern (Weaver 1954, Coppock 1966). Hence, a brief analysis of the ranking of crops provides a good summary of the regional dominance of crops and changes in the cropping pattern.

Aman rice undoubtedly occupies a paramount position in the cropping pattern of Bangladesh. In 1970-71, *Aman* rice occupied first rank in every district, except Chittagong HT and Kushtia, where it was superseded by *Aus*. In the final year of this analysis, despite a slight drop in the areal strength of *Aman*, it continued to occupy first rank in all districts except Kushtia (Table 3.6). Even in Chittagong its strength improved and it became the leading crop in the cropping pattern. *Aus*, which was the leading crop in Chittagong HT, was pushed down to the second rank. Thus, the regional pattern of the first ranking crop is very simple, it is *Aman* all the way. However, there is considerable variation in the density of *Aman* rice within the broad area where *Aman* is a first ranking crop. In some districts, *Aman* is first ranking with over half the TCA, but in some others it assumes first rank with less than a third of the TCA.

Aus rice, similarly, dominates the pattern as second ranking crop, with only a few exceptions. Only in three districts in the base year was it not the second leading crop, only because it occupied higher ranks in two and in one it was superseded by *Boro*. In the final year of the analysis, *Boro* rice assumed second rank in four districts where *Aus* was pushed down to the third position. The emergence of *Boro* rice as a second leading crop in four districts is an interesting development and is attributable to the expansion of irrigation and the introduction of HYV seeds.

Table 3.6
Ranking crops in Bangladesh

	Crop Ranks 1972-74 Avg.			Crop Ranks 1990-92 Avg.		
	I	II	III	I	II	III
Chittagong	A	Au	B	A	B	Au
Chittagong HT	Au	A	B	A	Au	B
Comilla	A	Au	B	A	Au	B
Noakhali	A	Au	B	A	Au	B
Sylhet	A	B	Au	A	B	Au
Dhaka	A	Au	J	A	Au	B
Faridpur	A	Au	J	A	Au	J
Mymensingh	A	Au	B	A	Au	B
Tangil	A	Au	J	A	Au	B
Barisal	A	Au	B	A	Au	B
Jessore	A	Au	J	A	Au	J
Khulna	A	Au	B	A	B	Au
Kushtia	Au	A	G	Au	A	J
Patuakhali	A	Au	B	A	Au	B
Bogra	A	Au	J	A	B	Au
Dinajpur	A	Au	J	A	Au	W
Pabna	A	Au	J	A	Au	W
Rajshahi	A	Au	B	A	Au	B
Rangpur	A	Au	B	A	Au	J
Bangladesh	A	Au	B	A	Au	B

Note: A= Aman, B= Boro, Au= Aus, W= Wheat, J= Jute, G= Gram
Source: Calculated by the author from BBS data

The distribution pattern of the third ranking crop is also significant as at least some of the third ranking crops make contiguous areas of appreciable extent. In the distribution pattern of third ranking crops, *Boro* rice stands out quite prominently as it occupies a large contiguous area consisting of Mymensingh, Tangil, Dhaka, Comilla, Barisal, Patuakhali, and Chittagong HT districts.

Jute is next in importance as a third ranking crop. It is the third leading crop in four districts, namely, Kushtia, Jessore, Faridpur, and Rangpur. The first three of these districts comprise a large contiguous area to the south of the Padma river. In each of the four districts, jute assumes third rank with less than 15 percent of the TCA. In four widely separated districts, *Aus* rice also occupies third rank. Although wheat occupies third rank only in two districts, it reflects an important change in the cropping pattern of Bangladesh. In the base year, the density of wheat was less than 2 percent in all districts with only three exceptions, but in the final year its density was well over 5 percent in at least 10 districts. So wheat is undoubtedly becoming an important food crop in Bangladesh and is beginning to make an important impression on the agricultural landscape.

The patterns of first and second ranking crops have changed very little. More noticeable changes occurred in the pattern of third ranking crops. However, most of the changes in crop rankings in Bangladesh appear to be related to the increases in the areal strength of *Boro* rice and wheat, two important winter crops. In some districts, the increases in the areal strength of *Boro* pulled it up from lower ranks to the third position. In some others, *Boro* moved up from third to second rank, and the third rank was occupied by the crop displaced from second rank as, for example, in Chittagong, Khulna, and Bogra districts.

The ten major crops, over time, have become more dominant in the cropping pattern, occupying larger proportions of TCA. In the base year (1970-71), the ten major crops occupied about 86 percent of the TCA but in the final year (1990-91) their areal strength had improved to 90 percent of the TCA (Table 3.6). The increased dominance of the 10 selected crops in the cropping pattern was due to the increased share of *Boro* rice and wheat in the TCA. While the proportion of *Aman* and *Aus* rice in the TCA declined that of *Boro* doubled. Similarly, the share of wheat in the TCA increased four times. Yet another notable feature of the changes in the cropping pattern is a decline in the proportion of pulses in the TCA collectively and individually.

Crop regions

A leading crop seldom, if ever, completely dominates the cropland. Often the domination of the cropland is accounted for by a number of leading crops. Identification of agricultural areas by single crop names has been widely used as, for example, the wheat region, the rice region or the jute belt. Such labels are often misleading as they do not portray a realistic picture of cropland use. Often the second and third ranking crops may be only slightly less important than the leading crop. The agricultural areas, therefore, should be named by crop complexes consisting of a certain number of important leading crops. Such a procedure will provide a more realistic picture of the cropping pattern in a given areal unit. However, the delineation of the leading crop complexes in a given areal unit is a complex problem. Weaver (1954) devised a very comprehensive procedure for the selection of the minimum number of crops that adequately represent the crop complex in a given area. Weaver's method has been successfully applied by some writers outside the USA. But his method does not always seem to work, specially in the Asian situation (see Dayal 1967). In this study, a very simple procedure similar to the one used by Dayal has been employed for the selection of a combination of prominent crops in a given area. The minimum number of leading crops that account for two-thirds of the harvested cropland or TCA are taken to be the most important and suitable for identifying a given area. For example, in Dinajpur district the first ranking crop is *Aman* rice, which occupies 50 percent of the TCA, and the second ranking crop is *Aus* rice, which occupies 23.5 percent of the TCA. The two crops together occupy more than 66 percent of the TCA. Hence, the most important crop complex in Dinajpur district is comprised of *Aman* and *Aus* rice. In some districts, one leading crop alone may account for two-thirds of the TCA, as *Aman* rice in Khulna district. In Khulna district, therefore, the agricultural landscape can be quite realistically identified by one crop, i.e., *Aman* rice. In some other districts more than two crops will be required to account for two-thirds of the TCA as, for example, in Dhaka.

The application of the above procedure produced six crop combination regions in 1970-71, the base year. The largest among them was the two-crop *Aman-Aus* combination region, which was spread over eleven districts (Figure 3.1). The *Aman-Aus* combination occupied one large chunk of area in the northwest and another in the southeast. The contiguity of the *Aman-Aus* region was interrupted by the three central districts, namely, Dhaka, Faridpur, and Tangil, where besides *Aman* and *Aus* a third crop jute was required to account for two-thirds of the TCA. These three districts formed the second largest crop combination region, consisting of three crops. The third largest crop region was the one-crop *Aman* rice region, occupying two coastal districts. The remaining crop regions in the base year occupied only one district each. They are the two-crop *Aman-Boro* combination in Sylhet, and the three-crop *Aman-Aus-Boro* combination in Chittagong HT, and the five-crop *Aman-Aus*-gram-jute-wheat combination in Kushtia.

In 1990-92, the final year, the number of crop regions increased from six to seven, suggesting some increase in spatial diversity in the cropping pattern. Not only did the number and boundaries of the crop regions change, but also the crops composing them changed. This clearly indicates that crop regions even in a largely subsistence agriculture, as in Bangladesh, are not static. They are dynamic features of the agricultural landscape.

In the final year, the largest crop region continued to be the two-crop *Aman-Aus* region, but with a considerably reduced area. The number of districts in this region dropped from 11 in the base year to 6 in the final year. In the majority of districts, where the combined areal strength of *Aman* and *Aus* declined to less than two-thirds of the TCA, it was due to increased areal strength of *Boro* at the expanse of *Aus*.

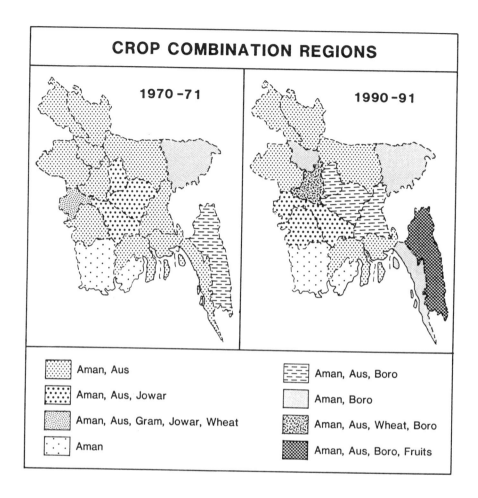

CROP COMBINATION REGIONS

1970-71

1990-91

Aman, Aus	Aman, Aus, Boro
Aman, Aus, Jowar	Aman, Boro
Aman, Aus, Gram, Jowar, Wheat	Aman, Aus, Wheat, Boro
Aman	Aman, Aus, Boro, Fruits

Figure 3.1   Crop combination regions

The second largest crop region in the final year was again the two-crop *Aman-Boro* combination, occupying three large but widely separated districts, namely, Bogra, Sylhet, and Chittagong. In the base year this crop combination region was found only in one district but in the final year it was spread over three districts. The two new districts that joined this crop combination region were Bogra and Chittagong.

The third crop region was the three-crop *Aman-Aus-Boro* combination, which occupied the central area of Bangladesh. In two of the three districts comprising the region, jute was replaced by *Boro* rice, and in Faridpur district *Boro* entered the three-crop combination by increasing its areal strength at the expanse of *Aus*. Due to reduced areal occupancy of *Aus*, *Aman* and *Aus* did not account for two-thirds of the TCA, requiring a third crop to be added to the combination.

The fourth crop region was the one-crop *Aman* region. It remained unchanged and occupied the same districts as it did in the base year.

The fifth region, in order of land occupancy, was the three-crop *Aman-Aus*-jute combination region, occupying three west-central districts. This region occupied more central position in the base year but has shifted to the western districts. The remaining regions are the two four-crop *Aman-Aus*-wheat-*Boro* and *Aman-Aus-Boro*-fruit combination regions, occupying single districts of Pabna and Chittagong HT, respectively.

The crop regions in Bangladesh are simple as they are heavily dominated by three varieties of rice. The rise of *Boro* rice, wheat, and fruits to prominence is noteworthy. The crop regions, although still dominated by rice, are changing significantly. In the base year, three-crop combination regions were found in eight districts but in the final year they were found in ten districts, indicating some increase in spatial crop diversification.

Summary

The agricultural scene in Bangladesh is dominated overwhelmingly by wet-rice cultivation, which accounts for 86 percent of the total cropped area. The ten major crops account for 90 percent of the cropped area, and with the exception of jute all are food crops. The areal strength of the ten major crops has improved over time. In the final year their share of the cropped area increased by 4 percent. *Boro* rice and wheat recorded the most prominent increases in their share of the total cropped area.

The crop regions have displayed some significant changes in the number of crops in each region. For example, some two-crop combination regions have changed into three-crop combination regions. There were three-crop combination regions in more districts in the final year than in the base year, indicating some diversification of agriculture.

4 Food production trends and potentials

To produce sufficient food from its own resources is a major concern of policy makers in Bangladesh. A careful scrutiny of the production of food crops, therefore, is essential to provide guide-lines for food production planning. This chapter analyses trends and future potentials of food production in Bangladesh.

Analysis of trends

Several writers have attempted to measure the growth of agricultural production (particularly foodgrains) in Bangladesh over different periods, using different methods and data sets. There are several important commonalities in the conclusions of these studies but there are also some notable differences.

Boyce used a modified data series to measure growth in agricultural output in Bangladesh over 1949-1980, 1949-64, and 1965-1980. He observed that before the introduction of the crop cutting surveys, official estimates of acreage and yield per acre of various crops were under-estimated. He supported his argument by comparing only acreage data in agricultural censuses with the annual estimates of acreage and average yields of crops published by the BBS. It appears that Boyce's observations were based on rather fragmentary evidence (Alauddin and Tisdell 1987). Further, his revised data series, particularly after 1965, are not very different from official series, hence not a significant improvement.

Boyce found that the annual growth rates over the three periods were positive but lower than population growth rates, except during 1965-80. His work also shows that annual growth rates of agricultural production, particularly foodgrains, have improved and the regional pattern of growth has changed over time. During 1949-1965, the southeastern districts displayed the highest growth rates, but during 1965-80, the growth was highest in the western districts. On the other hand, growth rates during 1965-1980 in Boyce's study are quite similar to the growth rates during 1971-91 derived here. For example, in both studies Bogra, Kushtia, Pabna, Rangpur, Dinajpur, and Jessore during 1971-1991 were fast growing districts, recording above average growth rates. Also, during 1965-80, in Boyce, and 1971-91, in my analysis, the growth rates for Bangladesh and for several districts were higher than population growth rates.

Using only official data and employing exponential functions, Hossain measured growth rates of foodgrain production in three separate studies, and found them higher than population growth rates (Hossain 1980, 1984, 1990). In all three studies, Hossain was quite optimistic about the growth of food production in Bangladesh. He believed that further expansion of irrigation would increase the area under HYVs and therefore foodgrain production.

Alauddin and Tisdell (1987) also used official data and critically examined the growth rates of foodgrain production in Bangladesh from 1971 to 1985. They used the same period as Boyce but also estimated growth rates for independent Bangladesh. The growth rates for independent Bangladesh were much higher than for any previous period, indicating that agricultural development and research were badly neglected during Pakistani regime. They believe that further spread of HYVs will certainly increase multiple cropping, if not yield per acre of major crops. However, they think that area under HYVs is not likely to increase very much, but they provide no evidence in support of their claim. In fact, they were wrong. The area under HYRVs increased much more than predicted by them.

Food production trends have been examined over a period of 19 years (1972-73 to 1990-91). The first two years of the 1970s (1970-71 and 1971-72) were excluded from the analysis because agricultural operations were somewhat disrupted by the war of liberation throughout the country, particularly in the major food producing districts in the north. After Bangladesh became independent, agriculture not only recovered rapidly from the devastations of the war but progressed much faster than during the pre-independence period.

The production and per acre yield data used in this analysis are quite reliable because the traditional subjective methods of estimation were completely replaced by objective methods of estimation, based on the crop cutting surveys, in Bangladesh by the mid 1960s.

Time series were constructed for acreage, production, and yield per acre of total rice, HYRVs, wheat, total pulses, and total foodgrains for the analysis of trends. Time series were also compiled for production and per capita availability of total foodgrains, sugar, gur, and meat. All data for the time series were obtained from various issues of the *Statistical Yearbook of Bangladesh* and the *Yearbook of Agricultural Statistics of Bangladesh.*

In this study, annual trends were computed for a period of 19 years by fitting linear regressions to acreage, production, and yield per acre data for selected food crops. Our assumption was that area, production, and yield per acre of food crops would rise over time, stimulated by increasing demand and improved technology. In the linear equations, annual acreage, production, and yield per acre of various crops were regarded as dependent variables (Y) and the time as an independent variable (X). The trend values were tested for significance by using t-tests and coefficients of correlation. Boyce employed an exponential function, which gives constant rate of growth, but provides no justification for his choice. Alauddin and Tisdell (1987) applied both logistic and linear functions to measure growth rates of foodgrain production and found that linear functions give better fit in terms of statistical quality of estimates. We have, therefore, used official data and employed only linear functions to measure the growth rates of foodgrain production in Bangladesh.

Changes in the production of foodgrains

Natural hazards (tropical cyclones, river floods, coastal floods, and droughts) often have devastating effects on the food supply in Bangladesh, creating a need for large imports and appeals for food aid. But despite the large fluctuations in food supply, the overall trends are quite encouraging. The foodgrain production in Bangladesh during the two decades (1970s and 1980s) increased at the annual linear rate of 421,200 metric tons or 3.97 percent (Table 4.1). This growth rate was significantly higher than the population growth during the same period. Hence, there was some increase in per capita availability of foodgrains.

Most of the increase in foodgrain production appears to have come from a large increase in rice production. Although the percentage increase in wheat production (150 percent) was much larger than rice, its contribution to the total foodgrain production was small because it was a new crop and occupied a much smaller area than rice — only 1.2 percent of the rice area. Hence, absolute increase in wheat production was nowhere near the increase in rice production. Rice production during the period increased by 84 percent, about the same as total foodgrains. As rice accounted for 95.5 percent of total foodgrains, it was undoubtedly the main source of growth in foodgrain production.

The annual average trend in rice production in Bangladesh during the reference period was about 380,000 metric tons or 3.84 percent (Table 4.1). Rice production increased from 10.6 million metric tons (1972-75 avg.) to 17.6 million metric tons (1989-92 avg.). Despite serious limitations on the expansion of agricultural land in Bangladesh, some increase in rice production did come from the expansion of rice acreage. It is very likely that much of the expansion of rice area came from re-cultivating *Boro* rice on the land that previously produced only one crop of *Aman* rice. Nevertheless, some expansion of rice area must have occurred on the new land, as during the two decades (1970s and 1980s), about 800,000 acres were added to the cultivated area in Bangladesh. This increase in the net cropped area came mainly from reduction in current fallow, therefore, the increase in arable land was only 30,000 acres during the period (FAO 1975 and 1993). However, increase in rice area relative to production was very small. While rice production in 19 years increased by 84 percent, its acreage increased by only 12 percent. Hence, the impressive increase in rice production was clearly attributable to increase in yield per acre indicating significant rise in productivity. The sources of increase in food supply in the post-independence period are strikingly different from those of the

Table 4.1
Production trends in selected food items 1972-73 to 1990-91

Growth measures	Rice Prod.	Yield	Wheat Prod.	Yield
Annual growth rates:				
absolute	379.300	24.700	72.700	56.300
Percentage	003.840	02.600	150.000	06.130
R^2	000.921	000.905	000.681	00.395
t values	014.100	012.760	006.100	03.480
Level of significance	.001	.001	.001	.003

Growth measures	Pulses Prod.	Yield	Foodgrains Prod.	Yield
Annual growth rates:				
absolute	8.900	-1.800	421.200	.250
Percentage	5.060	-0.270	3.970	0.160
R^2	0.604	0.065	0.944	0.003
t values	5.190	-1.480	16.980	1.020
Level of significance	.001	.158	.001	.321

Note: Production is in thousand metric tonnes and yield is in lbs. per acre
Source: Calculated by the author from BBS data

pre-independence period. During the 1950s and 1960s, for example, acreage expansion was the main source of increase in foodgrain production. The acreage expansion was due to expansion of cultivated land into new areas and increased frequency of cropping over existing cultivated land. After 1971, the situation changed dramatically. Rapid increase in already high rural population densities made expansion of cultivated land almost impossible. Attention was then focused more on improving productivity through raising average yields and intensity of cropping. The Government of Bangladesh played an important role in boosting food production. They gave high priority to the attainment of self-sufficiency in food supply, and allocated large funds for the expansion of irrigation, water control, and agricultural research in order to increase food production. This strategy proved quite successful and led to a strong growth in output. Increase in the average yield of crops became the main contributor to higher growth in foodgrain production. Between 1970 and 1992, the cultivated area increased little but production increased very substantially. Hossain (1984) estimated that 70 percent of the increase in output in independent Bangladesh was due to growth in average yields and some might have been due to a rise in agricultural intensity. The yield per acre of all rice (*Aman, Boro, and Aus*) including HYRVs during the reference period increased at an annual average trend rate of 2.6 percent (Table 4.1). The increase in the average rice yields in Bangladesh during the 1980s was so impressive that it made a noticeable impact on the average rice yield in Asia (Rosegrant and Svendsen 1993). Much of this impressive increase in average yield of rice is attributable to the adoption of HYRVs. Although the adoption of HYRVs in Bangladesh has not been very impressive, for all varieties of rice, relative to most other major rice producers of Asia, they have, nevertheless, made an important positive impact on the average rice yields. At present almost 90 percent of the area sown to *Boro* rice and 31 percent of transplanted *Aman* (T. *Aman*) are under HYRVs. In the early 1970s, it was suspected that *Aman* rice would not benefit as much from the HYRVs as other varieties of rice, but it has already been proved wrong. The percentage of *Aman* rice area under HYRVs is now larger than the area under HYV *Aus*. Despite considerable expansion of HYRVs, the increase in the average yield of rice was significantly lower than the increase in rice production, indicating that the additional increase in production came from higher intensity of cropping.

The increase in the area and average yield of wheat also made a significant contribution to increased food supply in Bangladesh. During the reference period, the area under wheat quadrupled and average yield doubled. Perhaps it would be difficult to find a parallel example of such a rapid increase in a major food crop anywhere in the world. Being a new crop, the contribution of wheat to the food supply of Bangladesh, relative to rice, was small but significant. In no other crop was the increase in area greater than production.

The production of pulses, which appeared to be declining during the 1970s, began to rise in the 1980s. It was reported in the Agricultural Census of 1983-84 that the area under pulses was under-reported prior to 1983-84 (BBS 1986). Therefore, decline in the production of pulses during the 1970s was not real because production is calculated from area and yield data. Post 1983-84 data for pulses are not comparable with pre-1983-84 data. Hence, it is not quite possible to work out accurately how the production of pulses changed during the reference period. Nevertheless, the revised data display significant positive growth in the acreage and production of pulses during the 1980s. An unusual aspect of the change in the cultivation of pulses, compared with other food crops, was that percentage increase in acreage and production were about the same, but the yield per acre declined (Table 4.1). One tends to think, therefore, that better land and inputs are being diverted away from pulses and into HYVs of rice and wheat. If pulses are becoming less preferred crops and receiving a neglected treatment, then this trend may have a serious effect on agricultural productivity and the environment in the long run. Pulses have been used in traditional agriculture to improve soil fertility through nitrogen fixation and have been an important source of protein in the diet of the common people.

Since independence, food production in Bangladesh has displayed strong growth, and consequently total food supply and per capita availability of food from domestic production have both consistently improved. The increased supply has not only raised average availability but also consumption levels of the poor, as indicated by Household Expenditure Surveys. The percentage of the population receiving less than 2,122 calories per capita per day — a level that is considered by many as the minimum requirement — has declined from 83 percent in 1973-74 to about 47 percent, which is similar to the percentage of the food poor in India. Whatever level of food intake one may take, one cannot deny that there has been an impressive progress in the elimination of hunger in Bangladesh during the last two decades.

The BBS constructs a annually published index numbers for several agricultural crops. In this section we have re-examined the changes in cereals, oil seeds, vegetables, and livestock and poultry — four main food items —using official production index numbers. Pulses were excluded because of the comparability problem of data as mentioned earlier in this chapter. All index numbers are for the base year 1972-73, which is the same as the base year for other data I have used in the analysis of trends.

From 1972-73, the base year of index numbers, to 1990-91, we have 19 years time series of index numbers, which expose some very encouraging facts concerning food supply in Bangladesh. One very notable feature of the selected components of food supply is that, despite some ups and downs, their production never dropped below the 1972-73 level during the 19 years, except for oil seeds in 1973-74 (Table 4.2) The increases in the production of rice (paddy), minor cereals, and oil seeds have been very impressive indeed, and have remained well above population growth. Hence, per capita rice output from local production in 1991 was 18 percent higher than in 1972-73 or at an annual growth rate of 0.95 percent. The increase in the production of minor cereals (mainly wheat) probably has no parallel elsewhere in the world. The output of minor cereals increased tenfold during the period.

Table 4.2

Index numbers of agricultural production, Bangladesh

(1972-73= 100)

Years	Cereals	Paddy all varieties	Minor cereals	Oil seeds	Livestock & poultry	Population	Per capita paddy
1972-73	100	100	100	100	100	100	100
1973-74	120	118	150	92	102	103	115
1974-75	118	112	129	104	103	105	107
1975-76	129	127	243	103	106	108	118
1976-77	119	118	295	107	105	110	107
1977-78	131	130	397	118	142	113	115
1978-79	124	129	563	122	148	115	112
1979-80	132	128	937	105	154	118	108
1980-81	142	139	1245	104	158	121	115
1981-82	148	148	1056	106	160	123	110
1982-83	148	148	1193	103	174	126	113
1983-84	148	148	1369	202	172	129	110
1984-85	153	153	1693	216	116	131	110
1985-86	155	155	1228	205	119	134	111
1986-87	159	159	1260	183	123	137	111
1987-88	160	160	1334	184	127	139	109
1988-89	162	162	1250	173	131	142	108
1989-90	183	183	1091	179	135	145	120
1990-91	188	188	1134	176	138	148	118

Source: Calculated by the author from BBS data

Livestock and poultry production also increased but since 1989 fell behind population growth. Nevertheless, in 1990-91 it was 38 percent higher than in 1972-73.

If we take increases in all components of food in Tables 4.1 and 4.3, it is quite clear that food supply more than doubled during the period, whereas population increased by only one and a half times. The production of cereals alone increased at an annual rate of 4.7 percent since 1972-73, compared with the population rate of 2.47 during the same period (Table 4.2).

The production index numbers provide yet another piece of evidence that despite population growth the per capita availability of food in Bangladesh has been steadily increasing.

Changes in the production of other food crops

Besides foodgrains, the production of fruits, vegetables, meat, fish, and milk increased considerably, particularly to meet the demand created by the rapidly increasing urban population, which increased from 6.6 percent in 1971 to 14 percent in 1991. The urban population with relatively higher incomes always creates large demand for fresh fruits and vegetables, leading to a large increase in fruits and vegetables (Table 4.3). The Household Expenditure Surveys conducted during the 1970s and 1980s show a substantial increase in per capita consumption of vegetables and fruits particularly in urban areas.

Table 4.3
Changes in the production of non-grain food crops
(000 metric tonnes)

	1972-73	1989-90	Percentage change
Fruits			
Mango	360	175	-51.2
Bananas	579	637	-10.0
Pineapple	68	157	130.0
Lichi	12	17	41.7
Coconuts	57	84	47.4
Jack fruit	189	254	34.4
Vegetables			
Pumpkin	67	64	-4.0
Brinjal	66	173	162.1
Potatoes	746	1140	52.8
Patal	17	20	17.6
Okra (*bhindi*)	7	10	42.9
Ridge gourd	15	18	20.0
Bitter gourd	17	17	0.0
Snake gourd	14	9	-35.7
Cucumber	13	14	77
Cabbage	35	63	80.0
Cauliflower	30	60	100.0
Water gourd	3	60	81.8
Tomato	52	85	63.5
Radish	63	158	150.0
Beans	20	33	65.0

Source: Calculated by the author from BBS data

The production of brinjals, cauliflowers, and radish, more than doubled during the two decades under consideration, and several other vegetables increased by more

70

than 50 percent (Table 4.3). A lot of small farmers prefer to cultivate vegetables rather than grain crops Because they take less time to mature and enable them to cultivate three crops in a year. Early producers of vegetables fetch high prices and make good profits. Many non-agricultural households, both rural and urban, grow vegetables for their own consumption and make a significant contribution to the total supply of vegetables, although their contribution does not enter into the official statistics. In the slum areas of Bangladesh, one can invariably see creepers of various gourds climbing on the thatched roofs of the smallest huts. Sometimes, small patches of land around the huts are also used for growing various leafy vegetables.

With the exception of mangoes, fruit production too has increased very substantially (Table 4.3). The pineapple production more than doubled. The production of other major fruits increased by more than 40 percent, except bananas, which increased by only 10 percent. Part of the increased fruit production is exported and therefore during the 1980s the value of fruits exported more than doubled.

Refined sugar output recorded an impressive 868.4 percent increase during the period. The per capita availability of white sugar more than doubled. In contrast, the production of *gur* (unrefined sugar), which is mainly consumed by the rural poor, declined by 4 percent during the period. The per capita availability of *gur* declined more than the total production because of the population increase during the period.

A very impressive performance for a densely populated country was that meat production more than doubled, and per capita consumption of meat increased by 45 percent. Likewise, consumption of milk, total and per capita, increased by more than 100 percent.

The above account of changes in foodgrains and non-foodgrain foods certainly sounds very encouraging. It suggests that not only total food supply in Bangladesh increased but there has also been an impressive improvement in the quality of the average diet. This conclusion is well supported by the results of Household Expenditure Surveys conducted in the 1970s and 1980s.

Regional pattern of growth

The analysis of regional data reveals marked regional variation in the growth of food supply. An outstanding feature of change was that the growth in production was far greater than the growth in cropped area in every district, again indicating, as in the national level analysis, very impressive improvement in productivity (Table 4.4). The most striking growth in both cropped area and production occurred in the western and southwestern regions of Bangladesh. The growth was relatively poor in the more densely populated eastern and northeastern districts. The production of foodgrains more than doubled in Kushtia, Jessore, Bogra, and Khulna districts and was equally impressive in Tangil and Faridpur (Table 4.4). The regional growth rates presented in Table 4.4 are higher than those arrived at by Hossain (1990).

Table 4.4

**Changes in the area and production of foodgrains
1972-75 to 1988-91 (Four year averages)**

Districts	Percentage change		Annual percentage growth rate	
	Area	Production	Area	Production
Chittagong	16.4	47.8	0.82	2.40
Chittagong HT	25.0	25.7	1.25	1.30
Comilla	-1.0	47.6	0.05	2.38
Noakhali	08.2	56.5	0.41	2.82
Sylhet	00.7	06.0	0.03	0.30
Dhaka	07.0	28.2	0.03	1.41
Faridpur	27.9	88.9	1.39	4.44
Mymensingh	04.4	54.3	0.22	2.71
Tangil	11.3	84.6	0.56	4.23
Barasil	09.6	12.4	0.48	0.62
Jessore	26.1	133.1	1.30	6.65
Khulna	19.8	130.4	0.99	6.52
Kushtia	30.7	155.3	1.53	7.76
Patukhali	29.7	62.1	1.48	3.10
Bogra	05.7	146.4	0.28	7.32
Dinajpur	42.8	50.3	2.14	2.51
Pabna	11.3	37.2	0.56	1.86
Rajshahi	13.8	55.0	0.69	2.75
Rangpur	12.7	64.3	0.63	3.23
BANGLADESH	15.9	60.85	0.97	3.38

Source: Calculated by the author from BBS data

This may be because Hossain's time series terminate at 1988 and mine extends into 1991. Further, Hossain used value of output and we have used quantity. Nevertheless the pattern of growth is very similar. Tangil, Kushtia, Bogra, Pabna, and Faridpur also stand out as high growth districts in Hossain's study. In the first four districts, the production of foodgrains increased at the annual average rate of more than 6 percent, which was much higher than the annual growth rate of Bangladesh. In Chittagong, Noakhali, Comilla, Dhaka, and Sylhet the growth rate of foodgrain production was well below the national average. In the remaining districts, food production grew at an annual rate of around 2 percent, with the sole exception of Barisal. Hence, in these districts, food supply lagged behind population growth. But the growth in the western and southwestern districts was so high that it more than compensated for the slow growth in the other parts of the country and kept the overall growth of food supply well above the population growth.

Faridpur, Barisal, Jessore, Kushtia, and Pabna districts, all located in the western half of the country, are among the leading producers of pulses in Bangladesh. Patuakhali, a wet and flood- prone coastal district, devotes considerable area to the cultivation of *Moong* and *Khesari* because they are cultivated in the winter season and are therefore not affected by floods. The cultivation of *Moong* is particularly concentrated in Patuakhali district, where the area under *Moong* per farm household is sixteen times higher than the national average (BBS 1986). The production of both *Moong* and *Khesari* almost doubled in Patuakhali during the reference period, while it remained the same in Faridpur and Barisal, the two other major producers of pulses.

Minor cereals, such as maize, jowar, barley, and a variety of millets constitute about 2 percent of gross cropped area and more than 2 percent of the total cereal production. Dinajpur, Rangpur, Pabna, Faridpur, and Rajshahi districts in the west are the leading producers of minor cereals. The western districts are quite dry in winter, and large areas are without irrigation, and therefore not suitable for the cultivation of rice or even wheat but are reasonably well suited for millets and sorghums. But in the more populated eastern regions of Bangladesh, social and physical environments both encourage relatively high yielding cereals such as rice.

Large areas in the western districts are low lying, and therefore retain enough moisture for a winter rice crop, without irrigation. Hence, there is notable regional concentration of minor cereals in the west. The production of minor cereals, unfortunately, has steadily declined during the period. For example, the production of barley, jowar, and maize in the year 1990-91 was only one-third of what it was in early 1970s. This trend will adversely affect the calorie intake of the poor, because minor cereals are less expensive than rice and wheat, and are mainly consumed by the poor. There are, however, large differences in the regional pattern of growth.

The regional variation in the growth of food supply is also clearly displayed by the official production numbers, published by the BBS. After 1984-85, the BBS stopped publishing production index numbers for districts, hence, the regional discussion is for 1984-85.

The production index numbers also portray a similar picture of regional growth in food supply as is presented by the acreage and production data of food grains. The most impressive increase in cereal production occurred in the relatively less densely populated western districts, namely, Khulna, Kushtia, Bogra, and Dinajpur (Table 4.5). In these four districts cereal production more than doubled. In Rangpur, Jessore, and Chittagong HT too cereal production increased well over the national average. Here again, a notable feature of increase is that in no district was the production level below that of 1972-73. This holds good even for the most densely populated and flood-prone districts. Hence, even at the regional level there is no evidence that population growth reduced the growth of food supply below the level of the base year. Only in four districts, namely, Sylhet, Barisal, Pabna, and Faridpur cereal production fell behind national population growth. Nevertheless, even in

73

Table 4.5

Table 4.5
Index numbers of agricultural production
for 1984-85 by districts

(1972-73=100)

Districts	Cereals	Oil seed	Fruits	Vegetables	Livestock & poultry
Chittagong	141	102	68	100	174
Chittagong HT	181	48	216	111	172
Comilla	161	410	76	197	164
Noakhali	149	128	92	89	181
Sylhet	121	56	62	128	178
Dhaka	130	105	71	96	172
Faridpur	127	152	115	223	174
Jamalpur	177	74	70	183	166
Mymensingh	156	54	65	250	175
Tangil	166	302	119	175	174
Barisal	108	121	218	78	181
Jessore	177	100	102	313	175
Khulna	236	138	86	225	188
Kuhtia	219	132	105	160	171
Patuakhali	123	315	207	119	193
Bogra	206	88	77	171	168
Dinajpur	192	81	66	176	176
Pabna	111	132	68	143	171
Rajshahi	147	101	33	149	175
Rangpur	178	58	66	86	17
BANGLADESH	156	113	94	140	175

Source: Calculated by the author from BBS data

these districts the level of cereal production was higher than that of 1972-73. In these four districts, the production increase was modest not because of population pressure but because these four districts are highly flood prone. In fact, the population pressure in these districts is less than the average for Bangladesh. These districts are high risk districts for investment, which is reflected in a relatively small area under HYVs.

Having established that the growth of food supply has been much higher in the western regions than in the east, the large regional differentials in the growth of food supply need some explanation.

In the western districts, the agricultural holdings are larger than in the eastern and southeastern districts and also larger than the national average. The per capita cultivated area is 20 to 25 percent higher than the national average and about 30 percent higher than in the eastern and southeastern districts. There is a marked concentration of small farms in the densely populated eastern and southeastern districts. In contrast, relatively larger agricultural holdings are concentrated in the western half of the country (Bangladesh Census of Agriculture 1983-84). Owners of larger holdings are more likely to afford the adoption of HYRVs because HYRVs require investment in purchased inputs. The adoption of HYRVs enables them to produce a larger surplus for which there is always a ready market in Bangladesh. But they are encouraged to produce a larger surplus only when prices are high enough to compensate for the cost of inputs. There is considerable evidence that farmers in Bangladesh agriculture do respond to price changes (Hossain 1990). Therefore, it would appear that relatively larger holdings in the western districts partially explain higher growth in food supply.

Some writers have argued that larger farmers invest less per acre in both labour and purchased inputs and cultivate land less intensively (Hossain and Jones 1983). They have suggested that higher output and better utilization of labour would result from redistribution of land with a view to creating viable peasant farms. Farm level studies have also demonstrated that small farms used more labour and practised higher agricultural intensity (Hossain 1977, Rehman 1980). This may have been true at one point in time a decade ago, but it does not seem to be true when we analyse food production changes. Perhaps it has changed over time due to the spread of HYRVs.

In recent decades, neither land productivity nor intensity of cultivation has been increasing as much in the densely populated eastern and southeastern districts as in the less populated western districts, where farms are relatively large and the level of agricultural intensity low. However, Comilla and Chittagong HT are two notable exceptions, where land productivity increased as much as in the western districts. As discussed in some detail in the next chapter, after reaching a certain maximum, agricultural intensity ceases to respond to further growth of population and demand in the densely populated small farm regions. Ali and Turner (1992), using village level data, also arrived at a similar conclusion. In the eastern regions of Bangladesh, which are very densely populated and have very small farms, the agricultural intensity levels have perhaps reached the maximum. The high growth in food production, therefore, has shifted from small farm eastern districts to western districts, where relatively larger farms and lower agricultural intensity provide greater opportunities for increasing production. Hence, high agricultural intensity is beginning to flow over into less densely populated large farm regions. The larger landowners, who may not have been responding to population growth in the past, are now motivated by market forces to produce more by using available land more intensively. It appears that they are now investing more per acre in productive improvements because they can make bigger profits by doing that, despite some government intervention. The government policy on the whole is to maximize food production.

The second variable that accounts for high growth in the western districts is greater expansion of irrigation in recent years. Irrigation facilities are expanding more rapidly in the western districts because, prior to independence, irrigation development was mostly concentrated in the eastern districts, namely in Chittagong, Comilla, Noakhali, and Dhaka. Therefore, western districts offered greater scope for irrigation expansion. For example, the highest expansion of irrigation between 1972 and 1990-91 occurred in Faridpur, Pabna, Dinajpur, Rangpur, Khulna, and Kushtia districts, where percentage of net irrigated area more than doubled. The expansion of irrigation in the western districts helped increase multiple cropping, yield per acre, and adoption of HYRVs.

Yet another factor that might have contributed to higher growth in the western districts is that, with a few exceptions, they are less prone to floods than the eastern districts. This makes investment in the west safer and more effective. The western districts for the same reason also provide a better environment for the spread of HYRVs, particularly for transplanted *Aman* (T. *Aman*).

Food production potential

We have already noted that the potential for expansion of cultivated area in Bangladesh is extremely limited. Land use data clearly demonstrates that cultivated area (net cropped area + current fallow + long fallow) has changed little during the last two decades. Some increase in the net cropped area was due to reduction in area under current fallow and tree crops. The harvested area, however, can be increased by increasing agricultural intensity in some regions through increased investment in irrigation. The expansion of irrigation will permit the cultivation of a second or a third crop during the dry but very mild winters, particularly in the western and northwestern districts. This will, however, increase the harvested acreage only marginally (Hossain 1980). It is, therefore, quite obvious that any further increase in food supply in Bangladesh must come from improvements in productivity. That is exactly what Bangladesh is successfully trying to do. During the reference period, the yields per acre of all major food crops increased very significantly, except for pulses. While the average yield of rice (all varieties) increased by 49 percent, the average yield of wheat increased by 116 percent during the period under review. The question, therefore, arises as to how much more can Bangladesh depend on the possibilities of increasing the average yields any further? What is the potential for increasing the average yields of major crops? To answer these questions one has to compare the average yield of crops in Bangladesh with those in other countries having similar social and physical environments. The yield per acre of rice in Bangladesh is among the lowest in the major rice producing countries of Asia (Table 4.6).

Scope for further spread of HYRVs

Since the mid 1960s, the introduction and spread of HYRVs have raised the average rice yields. The future average rice yield in Bangladesh, therefore, will certainly

Table 4.6
Yield per acre of rice (paddy) and wheat
in selected Asian countries in kg/Hc
1991

Countries	Rice	Wheat
Bangladesh	2612	1676
China	5663	3151
India	2629	2274
Indonesia	4351	-
Philippines	2825	-
Viet Nam	3086	-
Myanmar	2733	904
Korea, S.	6035	-
ASIA	3582	2372

Source: FAO Production Yearbook 1991

depend upon the spread of HYRVs. Regional environmental variables, such as irrigation, soil and terrain quality, and liability of land to floods and droughts, strongly influence the pattern of adoption of HYRVs. Applying a modified logistic model to Bangladesh data, Bera and Kelley (1990) estimated that the highest limit of adoption of presently known HYRVs for T. *Aman* has already been reached in Bangladesh. They argued that until new HYRVs were developed for drought and flood-prone areas of Bangladesh the adoption level was not likely to rise any further. Their analysis was based on data only up to 1985, when less than 20 percent of the *Aman* area was under HYRVs. More recent data for the last five years of the 1980s already seem to invalidate the results of Bera and Kelly's analysis. Between 1986 and 1990, the productivity in rice cultivation increased more rapidly than during any comparable period in Bangladesh. This exceptional increase in the average yield and production was, at least partly, due to a further increase in the area under HYRVs, assisted by the expansion of minor irrigation projects. During the last 5 years of the 1980s, the HYRVs area under T. *Aman* recorded a substantial increase (Table 4.7). While the HYRVs area under *Boro* increased by 77.5 percent, the HYRVs area under T. *Aman* increased by 49.8 percent, an impressive increase indeed. In the year 1989-90, 31 percent of the T. *Aman* crop was under HYRVs, which was 5 percentage points higher than the upper limit suggested by Bera and Kelly. It is important to note that this increase has occurred without any significant development of new HYRVs to suit drought or flood-prone areas.

Although HYRVs and other improved agricultural practices were introduced in Bangladesh during the 1960s, when the country was under Pakistan, more serious development efforts in agriculture were clearly made only after independence. In

1971, less than 7 percent of the *Aman* area was under HYRVs, but within 10 years after independence, about 20 percent of the *Aman* crop was under HYRVs. At the end of the next 10 years, 31 percent of the crop was under HYRVs. Clearly, the rate of growth of HYRVs under *Aman* during the second 10 years was higher than the first ten years. Based on the adoption rate of HYRVs, one has to be optimistic about further spread of HYRVs in Bangladesh. Greater adoption of HYRVs will of course be constrained by inadequate irrigation, particularly in winter in the western region, and lack of flood control in the low lying areas.

Measurement of potential rice production

The average yields of both rice and wheat in Bangladesh are below the average for Asia and far lower than Japan, China, Indonesia, Viet Nam, and South Korea (Table 4.6). Even if we exclude Japan, Korea (North and South) and China, which have temperate climates and more favourable cloud cover for photosynthesis to occur, the average rice yields in Bangladesh are still far below Indonesia, Viet Nam, and the Philippnies, which have somewhat similar environments (Table 4.6).

There are very noticeable differences in the average rice yields among the Asian countries. The countries that are outside the humid tropics such as Japan, Korea, and China have higher average yields than the countries in the humid tropics. Chang (1968) argues that these differences are due to agro-climatic variations. The flowering and fruiting of several plants are affected by the amount of sunshine received at a place, which is a function of latitude and length of day. The process of photosynthesis uses visible sunlight to produce carbohydrates. The rate of this process increases with increasing solar radiation to a certain point, but after this point any further increase in solar radiation does not lead to increased photosynthesis. Further, seasonal and daily temperature variations, which characterize the middle and higher latitudes and are practically absent in the tropics, exert an important influence on the formation and development of grains (Chang 1968). Relatively cooler nights and lower temperatures in the middle latitudes help transport carbohydrates to the grains, producing higher weight.

The International Rice Research Institute (IRRI) carried out an experiment to determine the maximum yields of rice in temperate and tropical environments. The participating farmers used the best known inputs, but those located in the temperate zones (Japan and southern Australia) obtained 78 percent higher yields than those in Malaysia and the Philippines, who also used similar inputs (IRRI 1965). Chang (1968), therefore, argues that rice yields in the tropical countries of Asia will never be as high as in Japan, north China, Korea, Australia, and southern Europe. He contended that rice yields in tropical Asia could not rise much beyond 2000 kg/Hc of paddy, Because constantly high temperatures, cloud cover, excessive moisture, and the lack of seasonality have a negative effect on the average yields. Several countries in the humid tropics in Africa, Central America, and Asia have already surpassed his 2000 Kg/Hc limit. In Bangladesh too, paddy production per hectare is now 30 percent higher than Chang's maximum limit (Table 4.6). In Indonesia, paddy yield is more than double the maximum limit suggested by Chang. It is, therefore, clear that Chang's conclusion suffered from some serious flaws. The question, therefore, arises, as to what potential yield we can take for Bangladesh in order to estimate the maximum future rice yields, and the extent of present regional departures from that target.

After a careful examination of per hectare rice yields in the humid tropical countries of Asia, it was decided to take the 1991 average paddy rice yield of Asia as the potential yield that Bangladesh can reach. It may be true that Bangladesh may never be able to reach the yield per hectare level of Japan, China, and Korea, Because of its more tropical climate, but there is no reason to suggest that it cannot reach the yield levels of Indonesia and Malaysia, which is more tropical than Bangladesh. We decided to be less optimistic and set the potential yield at 2,000 lbs per acre of clean rice, which is 8 percent lower than the current average rice yield of Asia.

Since agricultural intensity is not responding to population growth in several densely populated districts in the east (see Chapter 5), it appears that the maximum limit of agricultural intensity in those districts has nearly been reached. As a consequence, future food production levels in most areas of Bangladesh will be almost entirely determined by the average yields of single crops, mainly rice and wheat. The yield data for rice and wheat for the 1970s and 1980s are quite reliable; they indicate that per acre yields of both rice and wheat (all varieties) have been steadily increasing over time. The yield per acre of rice increased by 49 percent during the two decades since independence. The annual rate of increase in rice yield is positive and highly significant ($R^2 = .905$). Comparing the current yield of rice with the rather modest potential of 2,000 lbs per acre suggests that the average rice yields (all varieties) can be raised by at least 30 percent above their present level. If the modest potential, set here, is reached in the near future, it will increase food production by more than 30 percent Because some increase will also occur in other foodgrain crops.

During the last two decades, the average rice and wheat yields rose largely due to the expansion of the area under HYVs. In Bangladesh, the HYRVs produce 33 percent to 63 percent more than traditional varieties, depending upon the local environments and the level of inputs used. In the 1980s, the HYRVs were producing half a ton of rice more per acre than the traditional varieties. The principal source of future growth in average yields, therefore, would be further expansion of HYRVs, which would demand greater irrigation facilities and fertilizers. For both irrigation expansion and greater use of fertilizers there is considerable scope in Bangladesh, because both are at a low level relative to other Asian countries. At present only 25 percent of the net cultivated area is irrigated but according to one estimate 76 percent can be irrigated (Ahmad and Sampath 1992). Water is one natural resource for which there is no shortage in Bangladesh. During the two decades under consideration, net irrigated area in Bangladesh, by all types of irrigation, increased by 84 percent. The largest increase was in tube well irrigation, which increased by more than 2,000 percent. Tube wells are now major sources of

79

irrigation, irrigating 20 percent more area than all other methods combined. This has happened because the main thrust of irrigation expansion programs is on small scale irrigation. Shallow tube wells are particularly suited to the Bangladesh situation because they draw upon underground water which is more than replenished during the rainy season. Much of the heavy monsoon rain is lost in the absence of adequate storage facilities, except for the underground recharge. Tube wells are less expensive than canal irrigation and more effective for the small farm situation.

Fertilizer consumption level in Bangladesh is among the lowest in the Asian countries, but it has been rapidly increasing, despite problems of inadequate supply. During the reference period, fertilizer consumption per acre in Bangladesh trippled. The International Rice Research Institute (IRRI) found that higher fertilizer doses do not increase yields in the same proportion and that the maximum difference between HYRVs and traditional varieties is at the lower level of fertilizer doses (IRRI 1977). This is promising news for the poor Bangladesh farmers, and implies that it is possible to increase rice production by increasing area under HYRVs without increasing fertilizer consumption to very high levels. It also means that the spread of HYRVs in Bangladesh may not be seriously constrained by the problem of short supply of fertilizers and low purchasing power of farmers if they are educated about the proper use of fertilizers.

At present, only 43 percent of all rice area is under HYRVs. The area under HYRVs for *Boro* is perhaps close to maximum, but for *Aman* and *Aus* it is still small and suggests sufficient scope for expansion (Table 4.7). The Bangladesh Rice Research Institute (BRRI) has estimated that 60 percent of the rice area can be brought under HYRVs. A cursory examination of the government food policy and progress in the spread of irrigation, fertilizers consumption, and HYRVs clearly indicates that the BRRI has set an achievable target. It also suggests that the modest potential per acre yield for rice set in this study is quite achievable.

Besides productivity increases, some increase in food supply can also be obtained from minimizing wastage. An estimated 8 percent of the foodgrain output is subject to after-harvest losses. Improvements in storage, transportation, drying of harvested paddy, winnowing and threshing methods can reduce wastage and contribute to the available food supplies.

A matter of serious concern that may reduce the future yield increases and therefore food supply is the declining trend of yield per acre of HYRVs (Table 4.8). The average yield of HYRVs during the last two decades declined by almost 25 percent. The maximum decline was recorded for HYVs of *Aus* and the minimum for *Aman* (Table 4.8). Between 1970 and 1990, the yield per acre of HYVs of *Aman, Aus,* and *Boro* dropped by almost 16 percent, 37 percent and 18 percent respectively (Table 4.8). Similar declines in the average yields of HYRVs have also been observed in India (Chakravarti 1976, Maskina, Singh, and Singh 1987). As a consequence, the regional association between the area under HYRVs and yield per acre of all rice has become weaker in recent years (Table 4.9). In the early 1970s the association between area under HYRVs and yield per acre of all rice was very strong

Table 4.7
Rice area under HYRV as a percentage
of all area under a rice variety

	Aman	Aus	Boro	All rice	All rice yield lbs/acre
1970-71	01.41	00.51	26.56	02.56	1003
1971-72	04.68	01.01	35.34	04.64	953
1972-73	09.77	02.26	44.70	11.06	935
1973-74	14.46	04.28	56.03	15.67	1075
1974-75	09.20	08.90	56.74	14.80	1028
1975-76	09.67	10.32	55.94	15.02	1102
1976-77	07.29	11.33	57.53	12.95	1061
1977-78	03.98	12.20	53.83	12.01	1154
1978-79	06.16	12.83	55.95	13.57	1133
1979-80	14.53	13.25	62.98	19.66	1119
1980-81	15.93	15.61	64.35	21.28	1201
1981-82	15.89	15.00	68.90	22.23	1163
1982-83	17.91	15.05	75.38	24.84	1198
1983-84	17.71	15.92	76.09	24.95	1227
1984-85	18.91	15.85	78.13	27.15	1276
1985-86	19.54	16.94	79.12	27.61	1290
1986-87	20.62	18.70	81.11	29.51	1296
1987-88	21.61	17.86	84.37	32.30	1382
1988-89	26.54	15.56	87.40	38.17	1356
1989-90	30.89	16.65	87.78	41.00	1375
1990-91	34.00	17.30	88.93	43.21	1390

Source: Calculated by the author from BBS data

at r=0.899, indicating that regional differences in the average rice yields could be largely explained in terms of area under HYRVs. The situation changed considerably in the late 1980s. The regional association between the two variables became much weaker at r=0.692. This indicated that HYRVs were not contributing as much to regional differentials in overall rice productivity as they did in the early 1970s. It also implies that in the 1980s in some regions high average yields of all rice may not be due to high acreage under HYRVs but may be due to considerable improvement in the yield of traditional varieties.

Table 4.8
Changes in yield per acre of HYRVs
over time

Years	Aman	Aus	Boro
1970-71	2125.8	2656.6	2777.0
1971-72	2229.2	2137.6	2436.3
1972-73	1424.9	2041.7	2469.4
1973-74	1920.6	2321.9	2221.5
1974-75	1733.1	1993.5	2005.0
1975-76	1760.2	1972.8	2063.1
1976-77	1721.3	1835.9	1970.3
1977-78	1983.8	1866.1	2049.1
1978-79	1589.8	1844.8	1865.6
1979-80	1739.2	1674.2	2110.4
1980-81	1415.6	1796.1	2162.5
1981-82	1568.2	1757.4	2273.5
1982-83	1562.7	1600.6	2276.1
1983-84	1652.7	1634.8	2154.9
1984-85	1681.5	1501.9	2231.9
1985-86	1541.0	1552.1	2152.8
1986-87	1660.7	1444.7	2167.9
1987-88	1538.9	1451.2	2125.8
1988-89	1547.2	1416.3	2064.0
1989-90	1775.7	1400.3	2136.4
1970-73 avg.	1926	2278	2561
1987-90 avg.	1621	1422	2109
Percentage decline between 1970-73 and 1987-90	15.83	37.58	17.58

Source: Calculated the author from BBS data

The average yields of HYRVs heavily depend on fertilizers and irrigation. There is considerable evidence from the USA and several other developed countries that the gains from the use of chemical fertilizers begin to dwindle after reaching a maximum. After this point the average yields increase at a decreasing rate (Peirce 1990, Pimental 1984). At the global scale, fertilizer use increased ten fold during the last 40 years, but it generated only threefold increase in foodgrain production (Ehrlich, Ehrlich, and Daily 1993). In the US corn production too, one can see a similar trend, where fertilizer use increased much more than corn output. In Bangladesh, rice production is already displaying declining gains from fertilizer use. This is clearly indicated by a steady decline in the yield per acre of HYRVs (Table 4.8). It has been realized that soils are loosing fertility as a result of lack of management and inadequate length of fallow period. The does not get enough rest to recuperate. It has become so poor in micro-nutrients that it does not respond to chemical fertilizers as much as it did in the past (Government of Bangladesh, The Second Five Year Plan, 1983). Although the causes for this decline are not well known, some probable reasons are discussed below.

The short term effects of fertilizer use are impressive indeed, but the long term effects are quite damaging to the soil and environment. Continued use of chemical fertilizers results in acidification of soils and leads to a decline in the humus content of the soil and makes it compact and impenetrable. Lack of humus makes soil less fertile and less responsive to chemical fertilizers. It loses its capacity to retain moisture and to convert fertilizers into plant tissues (Alauddin and Tisdell 1987). Chemical fertilizers also displace other favourable minerals from the soil through leaching (Oelhaf 1978). It has also been observed that with time HYV plants become more susceptible to plant diseases and produce less per unit of land. Hence, soil becomes less productive and requires higher doses of fertilizers to maintain yields.

Further, when HYRVs were first introduced, they were planted in the areas that provided the best environment for their cultivation. Consequently the yields per acre were very high. Later, as the area under them expanded they were pushed into less favourable areas, resulting in comparatively lower yields. Also, when HYRVs were first introduced they were probably given proper doses of fertilizers, but as the area under them increased, farmers began to apply smaller doses because that is what they could afford. In the 1970s and 1980s, fertilizer prices have increased faster than rice prices, putting pressure on farmers to save on inputs.

The declining yields of HYRVs will impose serious constraints on food supply sometime in the future. Not all rice areas can have adequate irrigation and water control development. The yield per acre of HYRVs, therefore, is bound to decline as HYRVs spread into less favourable areas. Despite declining per acre yields of HYRVs, it is entirely possible that the potential yield per acre of rice (all varieties) set here will be reached because it is set at a low level relative to other Asian countries. The government is making all-out efforts to bring at least 60 percent of the rice area under HYRVs by promoting the construction of irrigation facilities, fertilizer factories, and rice mills. Besides the BRRI, large and small farmers alike are continuously carrying out experiments to find out the best alternatives (IRRI 1965).

Table 4.9

Regional association between acre yield of all rice and area under HYRVs in 1972-75 and 1987-90 averages

(yields in lbs per acre)

Districts	All rice yield 1972-75	HYRVs area as 1972-75	All rice yield 1987-90	HYRVs area as 1987-90
Chittagong	1344	50.83	1589	79.45
Chittagong H.T.	1321	41.31	1310	76.45
Comilla	1167	23.16	1389	57.70
Noakhali	893	27.26	1180	41.68
Sylhet	1016	13.80	1112	28.55
Dhaka	931	18.38	1282	42.23
Faridpur	659	2.35	858	14.70
Kishoreganj	976	23.89	1570	56.75
Mymensingh	985	17.41	1275	42.56
Tangil	864	11.32	1274	39.47
Barisal	823	13.13	807	13.00
Jessore	787	6.10	1357	39.20
Khulna	812	7.10	1135	16.22
Kushtia	821	8.79	1209	34.60
Patuakhali	742	6.49	902	04.44
Bogra	914	12.75	2031	65.52
Dinajpur	937	7.40	1219	30.08
Pabna	720	5.43	1276	37.37
Rajshahi	837	7.78	1512	15.27
Rangpur	915	8.05	1373	39.59
BANGLADESH	907	14.25	1371	51.18

Regional association

Correlation between Column (2) and (3) r=0.899
Correlation between   "   (4) and (5) r=0.692

Source: Calculated by the author from BBS data

Potential of other crops

The large increases recorded by several food crops, other than rice, clearly indicate that there is considerable potential for increasing their share in the food supply. The production of several foodgrains such as *Boro* rice, wheat, barley, gram, *masur*, *khesari*, potatoes, and winter vegetables will increase considerably with the expansion of irrigation. The output of these crops will be more reliable than *Aman* and *Aus* rice because they are cultivated during the winter season, when crop damage from natural disasters is relatively small. The per acre yields of several of these crops are also, like rice and wheat, lower than in comparable countries. Because they have a shorter growing season and they fetch higher prices than foodgrains, they have great potential.

Regional food production potential

There are considerable regional differences in the average acre yields of rice and also in the adoption of HYRVs and therefore in food production potentials (Table 4.10). With the exception of Bogra, the current average yields of rice (all varieties) are well below the potential of 2,000 lbs per acre. The current yields of rice in Bogra, Chittagong, Kishoreganj, Rajshahi, and Comilla are more than 70 percent of the potential, and in each of them the percentage area under HYRVs is close to or above the 60 percent target set by the government, except for Rajshahi (Table 4.10). In Rajshahi, actual yields are 76 percent of the potential but area under HYRVs is only 15 percent. There are several such districts, where actual acre yields are 60 percent of the potential but the area under HYRVs is quite small. As, for example, in Pabna, Rangpur, Dinajpur, Kushtia, Jessore, Tangil, and Dhaka, the average rice yields are 60 percent or more of the potential but area under HYRVs is substantially below the target. In these districts, there is maximum potential for increasing average rice yields.

Instability in food supply

The production of foodgrains, fruits, vegetables, and meat over the last 20 years, as demonstrated in the previous chapter, clearly displays that the food supply in Bangladesh has been consistently increasing (Table 4.11). This is confirmed by the positive slopes of trend lines for the above items. But the annual figures also clearly show that the domestic food supply in Bangladesh is subject to considerable annual fluctuations. This instability in food supply is a matter of serious concern as it escalates hunger in the country from time to time.

Factors affecting instability

In Bangladesh food supply is badly affected by the frequency and magnitude of floods, cyclones, and droughts. Although it is impossible to isolate weather effects from other effects on food production instability, the crop damage data provide some

Table 4.10

Rice production potential: yield of all rice varieties in lbs per acre compared with potential yield of 2,000 lbs per acre

Districts	Rice yield 1987-90	Rice yield percent of potential	Percent of rice area under HYRVs
Category I			
Bogra	2032	101.60	65
Chittagong	1589	79.45	80
Kishoreganj	1570	78.85	57
Rajshahi	1512	75.50	15
Comilla	1389	69.45	58
Category II			
Rangpur	1373	68.65	40
Jessore	1357	67.85	39
Chittagong H.T.	1310	65.50	76
Dhaka	1282	64.10	42
Pabna	1276	63.80	37
Mymensingh	1275	63.75	43
Category III			
Tangil	1274	63.70	39
Dinajpur	1219	60.95	30
Kushtia	1209	60.45	35
Noakhali	1180	59.00	42
Khulna	1135	56.75	16
Category IV			
Sylhet	1112	55.60	29
Jamalpur	1103	55.15	41
Patuakhali	902	45.10	4
Faridpur	858	42.90	15
Barisal	807	40.35	13
Bangladesh	1371	68.55	51

Source: Calculated by the author from BBS data

understanding of the effect of weather on instability. Bangladesh sits on one of the world's largest river deltas. It is a vast flood plain, interlaced by the Ganga,

Brahamaputra, and Padma rivers and their many tributaries. Every year, during the monsoon season, rivers overflow their banks and submerge large areas. It is hard to believe that in such a region lack of soil moisture also frequently destroys crop production. Nevertheless, it is true, and is due to extreme inequality in the distribution of rainfall over the year. Most of the rainfall comes during the three or four monsoon months, leaving the rest of the year mostly dry. Furthermore, monsoon rains are characterized by a high degree of uncertainty in the timing and amount of rainfall, which are most important weather elements that affect crop damage. In some years, the monsoon rains may come early and in some too late. Similarly, in some years rains may end too early or may persist too long. The timing of rainfall is important for planting and harvesting of crops. Therefore, the

Table 4.11

Changes in production instabilities in rice and wheat

Period	Crop	Coefficient of variation	Mean	SD
1972-81	Aman	11.8	6,805,000	803
	Aus	12.4	2,895,000	358
	Boro	14.1	2144,000	302
	HYV Aman	43.8	1,195,000	523
	HYV Aus	48.9	667,000	331
	HYV Boro	21.9	1,558,000	337
	Wheat	93.2	361,000	337
1982-92	Aman	9.6	8,040,000	771
	Aus	10.5	2,889,000	304
	Boro	24.2	4,359,000	1056
	HYV Aman	31.2	2608,000	813
	HYV Aus	17.5	858,000	150
	HYV Boro	28.9	3886,000	1125
	Wheat	14.6	1078,000	158

Note: Mean values are in metric tons

Source: Calculated by the author from BBS data

87

delay or early start of the monsoon rains adversely affects production just as does a prolonged or early end. The magnitude of monsoon rains is even more important because it may cause heavy floods or inadequate depth of water in the paddy fields, which may prevent growth. The damage by cyclones and droughts is relatively infrequent, but sometime quite substantial. In some years, it may exceed the damage by floods, as for example in the 1980s.

Until quite recently, the fluctuations in cereal output were the result of weather-related variables, described above, but lately the instability of food supply appears to have increased due to expansion in the cultivation of HYVs, which are more susceptible to damage from floods, droughts, and plant diseases. There is greater damage to HYVs during droughts because they need more water to benefit from fertilizers. During floods, HYVs get submerged even in low floods because they are dwarf.

At the national scale, the production instability for major cereals (*Aus* rice, *Aman* rice, *Boro* rice, and wheat) was measured for the period between 1971-72 and 1990-91, using BBS data obtained from various issues of *Statistical Yearbook of Bangladesh*. The coefficient of variation — percentage deviations from the mean — for Bangladesh was 19.16.

The national instability in food supply is high and makes food planning difficult indeed. On an average, Bangladesh imports less than 8 percent of the food requirements, but the import needs often jump to more than 20 percent of the requirements. This happens when the domestic supply may drop, say, by 15 percent in a certain year, which is not very unusual. Since such situations occur without any advance warning, it becomes extremely difficult to procure additional food either by importing it or getting it in aid. Reduced crop output causes serious problems for the small farmers and landless agricultural labourers. Small farmers have no reserve stock and they produce hardly enough for their own needs. Therefore, even a small drop in output causes hunger for them. Drop in output means less employment for the landless and higher market prices of food. Higher prices and reduced employment opportunities reduce the entitlement of the rural poor, causing hunger. Thus instability in food supply is a major cause of frequent widespread hunger in Bangladesh.

In order to examine changes in food production instability over time, the entire 20 year period —1971-72 to 1990-91— was divided into two 10 year components, i.e., 1971-72 to 1980-81 and 1981-82 to 1990-91. Contrary to expectations, the production instability of total cereals remained unchanged over time, despite considerable spread of HYVs during the 1970s and 1980s. By the end of the 1970s only 21 percent of all rice area was under HYRVs, but by the year 1991 the corresponding percentage was twice as high. This suggests that the spread of HYVs did not make any difference to the instability of cereal production thus far. Murshid (1986) also came to the same conclusion, although he used a different 20 year time series which ended in the year 1979-80. One may be tempted to think that weather conditions during the second decade were more stable and compensated for the increased instability due to larger area under HYVs. But crop damage data do not support that view. Crop damage due to natural calamities was about the same during the two decades. The instability of total production of *Aman* and *Aus* in the 1980s was slightly lower than in the 1970s, but that of *Boro* increased (Table 4.11). It appears that instability in total production of *Aman* and *Aus* is declining over time.

An examination of production instability for HYVs of rice and wheat leaves no doubt that HYVs suffer from much greater instability and will make total production more unstable some time in the future. In both decades the instabilities for HYV production were much higher than for total production of each variety of rice (Table 4.11). It is interesting to note that, like total production, instabilities for HYVs of *Aman* and *Aus* declined in the 1980s, compared with the 1970s, but that for HYVs *Boro* increased. This could be due to greater attention to flood control and other projects, which benefited *Aman* and *Aus* more than *Boro*. The work on these projects, which were greatly neglected before independence, started in the 1970s but it began to yield benefit only in the 1980s. Hence rain-fed crops, like *Aman* and *Aus*, became slightly more stable. Further, HYVs covered only small areas of *Aman* and *Aus* acreage in the 1980s (Table 4.7). By comparison, HYVs spread very rapidly in *Boro* and covered almost 90 percent of the crop by 1990. During the 1970s and 1980s, there was considerable expansion of irrigation , which helped the spread of HYVs of *Boro* rice — a dry season crop. Therefore, instability for total and HYV Boro production increased. Although HYVs suffer from greater instability, it appears that their effect on total production does not show when they cover only a small area. Initially, when the HYVs area is small, despite greater instability their reduced production in some years may still be comparable to traditional varieties. It seems that when the dominant portion of the output begins to come from HYVs, the higher instability of HYVs begins to show in total production as well. For example, the instability of total production of *Boro* in the 1970s was only slightly higher than the instability of *Aman* and *Aus*, but in the 1980s, when more than half the output of *Boro* rice began to come from the HYVs, the instability of total *Boro* production increased considerably, and was more than twice as high as the instability for *Aman* and *Aus*.

The data presented in Table 4.11 also exposed some more characteristics of production instabilities of cereal crops. Among the three rice varieties, the total production instability is the lowest for *Aman* and the highest for *Boro* in both decades. Again, the explanation is to be found in the production accounted for by HYVs. The contribution of HYVs to Boro production is far greater than in the case of *Aman* and *Aus*. For example, in 1971-72 the contribution of HYV to total production of *Aman*, *Aus*, and *Boro* was 12, 5, and 55 percent respectively, and in 1990-91 it increased to 46, 27, and 92 percent respectively.

The production instability for wheat presents yet another puzzle. Wheat is a new crop in Bangladesh, and from the beginning it was almost 100 percent HYV. In the 1970s, the production instability for wheat was very high (CV=93.2), but in the 1980s it dropped to a very low level. The coefficient of variation for wheat in the 1980s was much lower than for HYV *Aman, Aus,* and *Boro*. In the 1970s, wheat production was very small. It was a period of experimentation, and therefore farmers might have made many mistakes in the selection of seeds, location of wheat fields, fertilizer doses, timing of irrigation etc. Also irrigation facilities were quite limited, and crops might have often failed in several areas due to lack of soil moisture. Hence, production fluctuated considerably. In the 1980s, irrigation had expanded quite substantially, and farmers might have learned by experience all the important skills of wheat cultivation. All these developments stabilized wheat production in the 1980s. A wheat crop needs much less water, and therefore a much higher percentage of wheat, compared with Boro, is unirrigated. It appears that HYVs of wheat do better than HYVs of Boro without irrigation. Hence, instability of wheat in the 1980s was lower than that of Boro.

Clearly instability is higher for some crops than for others. For example, predominantly rain-fed *Aus* and *Aman* would appear to be more susceptible to the amount and timing of rainfall. However, the rice strains of *Aus* and *Aman* have become well adapted to their environment and successfully resist considerable departures from the normal. *Boro* rice and wheat, which are both cultivated during the same relatively dry season and depend more on irrigation, would appear to be less susceptible to rainfall variation. It may be noted that 20 percent of Boro and 60 percent of wheat are not irrigated, and therefore the magnitudes of both monsoon and winter rains are important for the cultivation of winter crops. Monsoon rain is important because soil moisture in winter is affected by it. In reality, production instability for *Boro* and wheat is much higher than the aggregate instability for cereals. Two reasons may partially account for higher production instability for the two crops. First, a very high percentage of *Boro* rice and wheat are under HYVs, which require much greater management of water and of plant diseases. Secondly, both wheat and *Boro* rice crops are affected by a larger range of natural calamities. They are often damaged by cyclones and hailstorms, which hit the country in March and April, as well as early floods in May. Also, because they are grown during the relatively dry season, even a minor departure of rain from the normal may cause much damage in non-irrigated fields. In contrast, *Aman* rice is damaged only by floods and rarely by droughts.

Regional pattern of instability

The problem of hunger is more serious in some local regions than in others. Therefore, for the purpose of food planning, it is important to identify the regional pattern of instability in food supply. We have examined the regional pattern of production instability at two different spatial scales, using district and *thana* level data. We calculated the coefficient of variation for total cereal production over the entire 20 year period. The aim of regional analysis was to identify regions of high and low instabilities. Hence, it was not considered necessary to break the 20 year period into two decades, as was done for instability analysis at the national scale.

The district pattern shows two distinct regions of high and low production instabilities. A large area in the west, consisting of Faridpur, Jessore, Kushtia, Bogra, Pabna, Rajshahi, and Dinajpur districts, suffers from high production instabilities — well above the mean — with Bogra, Kushtia, and Jessore occupying the top three ranks in the group (Table 4.12). A second large area — running in a north-south direction — consisting of Mymensingh, Dhaka, Comilla, Noakhali, and Chittagong districts, is distinctly a low instability zone. In the remaining districts, intermediate levels of instability prevail.

Districts in Bangladesh are fairly large spatial units, and therefore conceal several details, which are revealed when we examine instabilities at the more detailed *thana* scale. For a more detailed regional analysis of production instability of foodgrains, I used data for each of the 57 randomly selected *thanas* for the period 1971-72 to 1983-84. More recent data for *thanas* was not available. The mean value of the

Table 4.12
Regional pattern of production instability of total rice, 1972 -1992

Districts	Mean	SD	Coefficient of variation	Ranks
Chittagong	780.8	79.3	10.2	18
Chittagong HT	108.6	25.8	23.8	4
Comilla	951.6	124.6	13.1	15
Noakhali	709.7	87.2	12.3	16
Sylhet	1095.0	156.0	14.3	13
Dhaka	743.9	89.8	12.1	17
Faridpur	505.6	109.3	21.6	7
Mymensingh	1938.8	257.4	13.3	14
Tangil	462.8	81.7	19.1	9
Barisal	693.6	114.0	16.4	12
Jessore	650.8	182.8	28.1	3
Khulna	596.6	114.3	19.1	9
Kushtia	257.0	81.1	31.5	2
Patuakhali	403.0	69.4	17.2	11
Bogra	626.5	237.5	37.9	1
Dinajpur	713.0	145.6	20.4	8
Pabna	407.3	94.0	23.1	5
Rajshahi	847.6	194.1	22.9	6
Rangpur	1283.6	230.3	17.9	10
Bangladesh	13774.7	2021.2	14.7	-

Note: Mean values are in thousand metric tons
Source: Calculated by the author from BBS data

coefficient of variation for cereal production for 57 *thanas* was 27. There are very notable regional variations in instability of food supply (Figure 4.1). It appears that production instability of foodgrains in Bangladesh tends to decline when data are

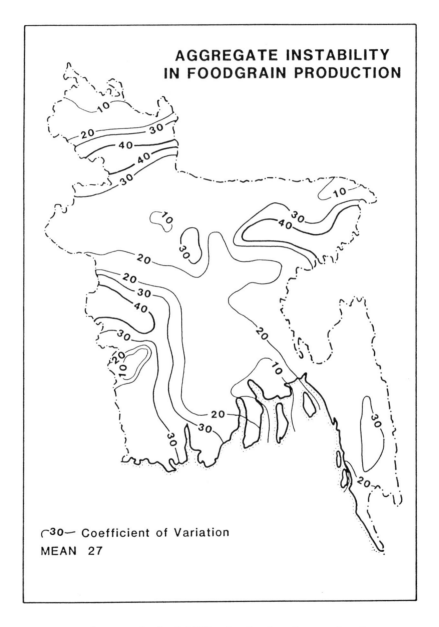

Figure 4.1 Aggregate instability in foodgrain production

92

aggregated. The mean of the coefficients of variation for *thanas* is much higher than for the districts and for the country.

In some local regions the instability of food supply is very high. For example, in the Sylhet basin, northern Brahamaputra flood plains and west-central districts, the coefficient of variation for cereals supply is 40 in several *thanas*. This means that in some local regions the domestic food supply sometimes may drop by 40 percent below the normal. This may trigger the development of famine conditions because food prices begin to rise, leading to hoarding of food by producers and wholesalers. The higher production instability in the western region - as revealed in both spatial scales — is probably due to higher concentration of HYVs of *Boro* and wheat in the relatively drier west. *Boro* rice, which is largely under HYVs, suffers from much greater instability than *Aus* or total foodgrains. In central Bangladesh, as revealed in the district analysis, the instability is low. This does not mean that the central region is less prone to natural disasters. On the contrary, the damage by natural calamities in this region is quite normal. The districts in this region are along the major rivers, which often overflow during the monsoon rains and inundate large areas in their vicinity, and do considerable damage to standing crops. Often more than 15 percent of the crops may be damaged by floods, droughts, cyclones, and hail. There are striking similarities in the regional patterns of cereal production instability based on the district and *thana* data, but the latter is more refined, therefore, more useful for food planning. For example, the instability for Sylhet is not very high, but some *thanas* within the district suffer from very high instability.

Food production policy

Government food policy will certainly affect attainment of the food production potential of the country. The food production policy of Bangladesh has the following main objectives: 1) to stabilize food prices for the consumer; 2) to provide minimum incentive price for producers; 3) to maximize food production in order to achieve self-sufficiency as early as possible; 4) to promote the development of winter crops, which are less prone to damage by natural hazards, and 5) to expand the irrigated area and the area covered by drainage and flood control schemes.

The government declares procurement prices at which the farmers can sell rice and wheat to the government purchasing centres. The government then releases the foodgrains to the public through ration shops, sales in the open market, and Public Food Distribution Schemes. The sales and distribution of foodgrains by the government in this way indirectly regulates availability and controls prices (Hossain 1990).

Although the government would like to provide maximum incentives to the food producers, it also has moral obligation to the poor. So, it tries to strike a balance between incentives to the producers and fulfilling the food needs of the poor. During natural disasters, the government, therefore, releases only half of the additional imports of foodgrains, through PFDS, in order to increase domestic supply only moderately to keep prices at a reasonably high level.

Some may argue that price incentives may not have a significant effect on production in Bangladesh because subsistence farmers, who dominate the agricultural scene, are not responsive to price changes. Those who hold such a view ignore the fact that even subsistence producers must generate some surplus above their own needs in order to have some cash income to buy essential goods that they don't produce on their own farms. Quasem (1987) reported that in Bangladesh 75 percent of the paddy producers sell a part of their output for cash income. It is now well established that farmers even in largely subsistence agriculture are responsive to price changes, and that the responsiveness has increased with the spread of the HYRVs (Alam 1992). In the 1980s, the market price of rice was found to be one of the two major factors affecting marketed surplus in Bangladesh (Quasem 1987).

There is limited scope in Bangladesh for developing a strong export oriented manufacturing sector Because the country is poor in energy, mineral resources, and also skilled manpower. It is unlikely that manufacturing exports, in the near future, will be able to pay for food exports, if agricultural development is neglected. The government, therefore, has rightly chosen to give priority to agricultural development in order to achieve self-sufficiency. This strategy is now considered superior to export oriented industrial development because of unfavourable global trade and financial environment (Baliscan 1993). Agricultural growth is expected to make the country self-sufficient in food supply and provide stimulus for non-agricultural activities (Bautista 1988).

An important aspect of the government food and agricultural development policy is to expand the area under irrigation, drainage, and flood control. As this segment of development does not attract private investment due to low returns, the government plays a major role in its development. Water control and management is the key issue in increasing food production in Bangladesh. From May to October there is so much water that about a third of the country is under deep floods and another one third under shallow floods. In contrast, from December to April, soil moisture is too low for crop production, except in some low lying areas. Therefore, drainage, flood control, and expansion of irrigation are essential for increasing food supply. The government allocated about a third of the total outlay of the second and third Five Year Plans for agriculture and water resource development. As a result, a quarter of the net cultivated area is now covered by drainage and flood control facilities and has irrigation. Considering the physical nature of the country and the structure of agricultural holdings, investment in minor irrigation projects has rightly received high priority. Development of minor irrigation has contributed immensely to the growth of winter crops notably *Boro* rice and wheat. In fact, the expansion of minor irrigation projects was the main source of growth in agricultural production during the 1970s and 1980s.

In Bangladesh, irrigated agriculture has been the focus of development but not much attention has been given to rain-fed agriculture, despite its much larger contribution to food supply. The relative neglect of rain-fed agriculture is because investment in it entails more risk. The crop damage due to floods, cyclones, and droughts is mostly during the rainy season. Nevertheless, rain-fed agriculture deserves more attention simply because it contributes more to the food supply.

A World Bank report recommends development of rain-fed agriculture, drainage and flood control, irrigation, and support services in order to realize full food production potential in Bangladesh (World Bank 1986).

Summary

Foodgrain production in Bangladesh, during the reference period, increased at an annual linear growth rate of 3.97 percent, much higher than the population growth rate during the same period. The growth rate of rice production was the most impressive among all cereals. Rice production increased from 10.6 to 17.6 million metric tonnes during the period. The growth rate of wheat production was even more impressive, but because of its small area its contribution to the total food supply remained small. The HYVs of cereals made a very notable contribution to the increase in food supply. But it is important to note that the HYVs also appear to be making the food supply more unstable. For example, the production of *Boro* rice, which has a very high percentage of total area under HYVs, has become more unstable than the production of *Aman* and *Aus*.

Besides foodgrains, the production of fruits and vegetables and some other food items such as meat, fish, milk, and sugar also displayed an impressive positive trend. Now several non-cereal food items are making an important contribution to the quantity and quality of the food supply in Bangladesh. Government policy played an important role in boosting food supply by investing in the expansion of irrigation, water control, and agricultural research. Employing an objective method, we have established that Bangladesh has the potential for increasing rice production by at least another 30 percent, using only existing technology and plant breeds.

5 Food production efficiency under increasing population pressure

Introduction

A vast majority of the population (85 percent) in Bangladesh is rural, and it is growing faster than in most Asian countries. The bulk of the burden of the rapidly growing labour force is borne by the agricultural sector because the non-agricultural sector of the economy is small and not expanding fast enough to absorb the growing labour force. Consequently, the rapid population growth has had a dampening effect on the agrarian structure in Bangladesh. Among the several changes, the deteriorating ratio of people to arable land is causing the most concern in the context of food supply. The worsening people/land ratio has led to a consistent decline in the average size of holdings and an increase in the number of small farms, fragmentation of farms, and landlessness.

The changes in farm structure can be examined more reliably since 1960 because of the availability of census data. Since 1960, there has been a steady decline in the average size of agricultural holdings and an increase in the ratio of people to arable land. The average size of holdings declined from 3.6 acres in 1960 to 2.3 acres in 1983-84 (Table 5.1). The rural population density on net cropped area increased from 2.53 per acre in 1965 to 4.4 per acre in 1990-91. Therefore, each acre of arable land is consistently required to produce more and support more people. This uninterrupted decline in the size of agricultural holdings tends to make several small holdings economically unviable. The process that makes farms smaller and fragmented is rather complex and needs some explanation.

If the size of a farming household continues to increase, a time comes when there will be far too many workers on the small holding. The family farm will not provide enough work for all members. Some members of the household will have to leave farm work and may become full-time agricultural labourers. Some others

Table 5.1
Changes in agricultural structure

	1960	1977	1983-84
Per capita cultivated land of farm households (acres)	0.37	0.26	0.25
Average size of holdings	3.60	3.50	2.30
Area and number of small farms, < 2.5 acres:			
Number (millions)	3.10	3.00	7.00
Area (million acres)	3.50	4.00	6.60
Area %	16.20	19.00	29.00
Medium farms (2.5 to 7.5 acres as percentage of all farms)	-	40.80	24.70
Large farms (> 7.5 acres) as percentage of all farms	-	9.40	4.90

Source: Compiled from *Bangladesh Census of Agriculture and Livestock, 1983-84*

may leave the village and move to cities in search of labouring jobs or small business opportunities in street trading. When the head of the household dies the small holding is subdivided among all the offspring, including those who left the farm for other income earning activities. Hence, the holdings of the offspring are even smaller than that of their parents. On such small holdings the inheritors will not be able to make a living and may be forced to sell. These small holdings are often bought by the large landholders because only they have money. This will lead to fragmentation of the holdings of the purchaser, who may have his initial plot at some other location. Also it is often the case that the members of one household may also inherit land from other relatives, who may die without an offspring. The holdings of the other relatives may be found at some distance from their own and sometimes even in another village. This process involved in the inheritance of land leads to further fragmentation of holdings.

Some small holders may continue to cultivate their holdings, but to make ends meet they may lease in some land from larger landholders or absentee landlords on a share cropping basis. Therefore, as farms become smaller, tenant farming also becomes more prevalent.

Due to changes in the definitions of terms and methods of enumeration, the data obtained from 1960, 1977, and 1983-84 agricultural censuses are not strictly commensurate. Nevertheless, some broad comparisons can be made. Between 1960 and 1983-84, a 24 year period, the number of small farms more than doubled, from 3.1 million to 7 million (Table 5.1). Also, the area under small farms nearly doubled. The percentage of total farm area in small farms increased from 16.2 percent to 29 percent of total farm area. The proportion of small to total farm numbers increased from 51 percent to 70.3 percent during the period. In contrast, the number of medium and large farms decreased over the period (Table 5.1). The number of large farms in a land scarce country has always been small, but it dropped further during the period from 10.7 percent to 7.6 percent of all farms.

The increase in the number of small farms and tenant farming may have two possible effects on food supply. The conventional economic theory of production suggests that a reduction in size will adversely affect production efficiency. This may happen because small farmers, who have little or no surplus, may not be able to afford the required level of yield augmenting inputs and therefore their output will go down. At the same time, they will not be interested in maximizing production on leased land because they know that half of the output will be taken away. They will, therefore, put in minimum effort on the leased land. Hence, according to this view, there will be a decline in productivity and a consequent drop in food supply. The second view is that small farms have a higher level of price and technical efficiency. This view is confirmed by extensive testing of farm level data from developing countries (Sen 1964, Khusro 1964, Lau and Yotopolous 1971, Yotopolous and Lau 1973, Hossain 1977, Rao and Chotigeat 1981, Taslim 1989). The argument in support of the latter experience is that because farmers on the small farms have no capital to buy more land, they substitute their own labour for capital. They work longer hours and harder in meticulous preparation of the fields, weeding, application of farm yard manure, lifting accumulated rain water manually for irrigation, and harvesting, and end up producing more per unit area than the large farmers. They also use a limited amount of land more intensively and use more irrigation and consequently have a higher total productivity (Singh 1990). Although there is some evidence that small holdings use more of all inputs per unit area, it is absolutely certain that they are more labour intensive. Abedin and Bose (1988) found that existing technology in Bangladesh is in favour of small farms and that if small farms were given equal access to inputs they may prove to be more productive even after the introduction of HYRVs.

In Bangladesh, post-independence production and average yield data of most food crops support the second view. The data clearly show that despite the declining size of farms, food supply has continued to increase at a rate higher than population growth. In Chapter four it was established that the average yields and total output of food crops consistently increased during the last two decades.

Food production efficiency over time and space

Food production efficiency may be defined in various ways. In a general sense, it denotes the efficiency with which resources - land, labour, and other inputs - are used in producing a given output of food. The most satisfactory measure of productivity, therefore, appears to be the ratio between the output and all inputs used in production, which is an overall measure of productivity. There are also single factor productivity measurements, which are concerned with the efficiency of individual factors. In this study we are concerned with the spatial and temporal comparisons of food output per unit of land and per agricultural worker.

The Bangladesh Bureau of Statistics (BBS) compiles value of total agricultural production (which is 96 percent food) and several of its components, which began to be published from 1976-77. The gross value is obtained by multiplying the quantity of output of each commodity by its market price. The value of production data are excellent for the measurement of food production efficiency per unit of land and per worker.

The BBS data on the value of agricultural production were extended backwards to the year 1972-73 — the base year in this analysis — for examining change. The data were then used for assessing temporal and regional changes in food production efficiency per unit of land in Bangladesh. However, serious problems were encountered in examining temporal and regional changes in food production efficiency per agricultural worker, because labour force data are not collected annually. Labour force data are collected during decadal population censuses and occasional Labour Force Surveys. They are available for 1974, 1981, 1983-84, and 1991. These data are, unfortunately, not comparable due to the changes in the definition and differences in the coverage. Only the BBS data on male agricultural workers, therefore, could be used for analysing temporal and regional changes in food production efficiency per worker. Fortunately, the Food and Agricultural Organization (FAO) annually compiles data for cereal production, arable land, and economically active population in agriculture. These data can be used for measuring changes over time in food production efficiency per unit of arable land and per agricultural worker. However, the FAO data are compiled only at the national scale and therefore cannot be used for regional analysis.

Food output per unit of land

The BBS and FAO data on the value and quantity of food crops respectively, clearly show that output per acre has consistently increased in Bangladesh, despite rapidly growing population and agricultural labour force. The BBS value of agricultural production (which is 96 percent food crops) per acre at constant prices increased by almost 61 percent over a period of 15 years, or nearly 3.2 percent per year, if we take the difference of the last three years average 1988-91 over the average of the first three years — 1972-75 (Table 5.2). The value of production, at constant prices, has been increasing at the rate of about 464 million takas per year since independence. The FAO data on the quantity of cereal production portrays a similar picture. The cereal production per hectare of arable land increased from 2.02 metric tons in 1972-73 to 3.21 metric tons in 1991-92, which represents an increase of again 60 percent over a period of 19 years or 3.2 percent per year (Table 5.3). During this period, the population in Bangladesh increased by 48 percent, and the economically active population increased by about 43 percent. Hence, quite clearly, food production not only kept pace with population growth, but actually surpassed it.

Sources of increase in food output per acre

In Bangladesh, the net cropped area and arable land have remained almost unchanged since independence (Tables 5.2 and 5.3). Hence, most of the increase in food supply

Table 5.2
Output per unit of land

Years	Value of agricultural production at 1969-7 prices (000 Takas)	NCA (000 ac.)	Value of output per acre of NCA
1972-73	11,653,156	20,840	559
1973-74	12,021,837	20,977	573
1974-75	12,390,518	20,559	603
1975-76	12,759,199	20,968	608
1976-77	13,127,880	20,445	642
1977-78	14,899,625	20,693	720
1978-79	16,838,910	20,801	809
1979-80	14,850,297	20,873	711
1980-81	16,170,246	21,158	764
1981-82	15,973,760	21,212	753
1982-83	17,488,546	21,369	818
1983-84	18,584,046	21,442	867
1984-85	19,752,898	21,353	925
1985-86	17,019,151	21,661	786
1986-87	18,064,601	21,878	825
1987-88	18,535,644	20,478	905
1988-89	17,798,373	20,148	883
1989-90	18,453,825	20,633	894
1990-91	20,460,519	20,198	1,013

Source: Compiled from the BBS data. NCA= Net cropped area

has come from increases in crop yields and agricultural intensity. The output of food per acre may be influenced by a number of interrelated factors, because the introduction of some improvements is often followed by several other developments. For example, the introduction of irrigation leads to greater use of fertilizers, human labour, HYV seeds, and higher agricultural intensity. Hence, it is impossible to determine precisely the contribution of each factor independently. For this reason, Dayal (1989) applied factor analysis to identify the sources of land and labour productivity in Bangladesh, using cross-sectional data. In Bangladesh, agricultural productivity is synonymous with food productivity, because out of 23 major crops taken by Dayal for measuring agricultural productivity, 21 were food crops.

Table 5.3
Food production efficiency measured in metric tonnes of output per hectare and per male agricultural worker over time

Years	Cereal production (000)	Cereal yield (000)	Econ. active population (000)	Arable land (000 Hc)	Productivity Land	Labour
1970-71	15090	1583	16701	8883	1.70	0.90
1971-72	15324	1555	16911	8900	1.72	0.91
1972-73	18023	1785	17142	8904	2.02	1.05
1973-74	17109	1690	17377	8921	1.92	0.98
1974-75	18655	1804	17615	8917	2.09	1.06
1975-76	17908	1769	17853	8912	2.01	1.00
1976-77	19762	1923	18094	8906	2.22	1.09
1977-78	19675	1900	18338	8915	2.21	1.07
1978-79	19902	1924	18586	8924	2.23	1.07
1979-80	21696	2004	18802	8913	2.43	1.15
1980-81	21589	1940	19182	8912	2.42	1.12
1981-82	22339	1996	19569	8863	2.52	1.14
1982-83	22847	2042	19965	8862	2.58	1.14
1983-84	23176	2147	20368	8863	2.62	1.14
1984-85	23995	2159	20704	8866	2.71	1.16
1985-86	24179	2162	21123	8895	2.72	1.14
1986-87	23372	2346	21550	8895	2.63	1.08
1987-88	24230	2304	22167	9000	2.69	1.09
1988-89	28795	2565	22681	9020	3.19	1.27
1989-90	29120	2491	23593	8853	3.29	1.23
1990-91	28320	2586	24087	8896	3.18	1.18
1991-92	28538	2640	24576	8894	3.21	1.16

Source: Calculated by the author from the FAO data

Dayal (1989) found that demographic pressure on agricultural land has had a positive influence on food output per acre. The output per acre was noted to be relatively high on small farms, in densely populated regions and where agricultural

101

intensity was high. The food output per acre was higher in the regions where small farms, high rural population densities, and high agricultural intensity overlapped. The interconnections between these three variables are well known. We have already stated earlier that increased pressure of population leads to smaller and fragmented holdings, compelling farmers into more intensive cultivation, in order to produce enough for subsistence. These three variables that have a positive influence on the output per acre, therefore, clearly demonstrate the farmer's response to demographic pressure. An important point brought out here is that food output can be increased by increasing the input of labour, which is a cheaper factor of production than land and yield - augmenting inputs. This relationship has also been established by others for Bangladesh (Chaudhury 1981, Gill 1983). The negative influence of farm size and positive influence of population pressure and agricultural intensity on output per acre direct attention to anti-Malthusian theories, that have drawn much interest and led to much debate in the literature on agriculture development (Brookfield 1962, Habakuk 1963, Boserup 1965, Clark 1967, Simon 1975 and 1977). These theories will be briefly reviewed later on in this chapter.

The factor analysis by Dayal (1989) also brought out clearly the point that irrigation, fertilizer use, and HYV seeds have a very important positive influence on food output per acre. These three variables are widely acknowledged determinants of output per acre in agriculture, and in Bangladesh they seem to reflect the influence of the Green Revolution. The Green Revolution has made a very important contribution to increases in food supply in independent Bangladesh.

The spatial pattern of output per acre is not very clear cut. High productivity, above the national average, is found in Chittagong, Chittagong HT, Comilla, Mymensingh, Jessore, Kushtia, and Bogra districts, which do not form a contiguous region. The first three are in the northeast, and the last three are in the west, while Sylhet occupies a northcentral location. In the lowest category of output per acre are Khulna, Patuakhali, and Barisal - three coastal districts - and Sylhet, a low lying district; these are all more prone to flood damage. Intermediate levels of productivity are quite scattered and do not display any significant spatial concentrations of a certain range.

There are very striking regional differences in the growth of food output per acre. The highest growth during the reference period occurred mostly in the less populated western districts — Rajshahi, Kushtia, Jessore, Bogra, and Faridpur, where the increase was well over 40 percent, and reaching 70 percent in some cases (Table 5.4). In the more densely populated eastern districts, only Comilla and Chittagong HT recorded high growth rates, above the national average. Hence, there appears to be a contiguous belt of high productivity growth that cuts right across Bangladesh from west to east (Table 5.4). The lowest growth was found in the coastal districts and Sylhet and Tangil, where the damage to crops from floods and tropical cyclones is the most severe. Sylhet and Tangil are both low lying districts and are heavily inundated during the floods. The coastal districts, on the other hand, face persistent damage to crops from winds and flooding from violent cyclones. In the remaining districts, the growth around the national average was minimal.

Table 5.4
Regional changes in land productivity between 1976 and 1991
(value of agriculture production at 1969-70 prices)

Districts	Production (000 Takas)		NCA (000 ac)		Land Productivity 1976-79 1988-91 Takas/acre		% Change
	1976-79 (3 years avg.)	1988-91	1976-79 (3 years avg.)	1988-91	1976-79	1988-91	
Chittagong	714,381	885,361	701	704	1,019	1,258	23.45
Chittagong H.T.	136,960	264,853	169	222	810	1,193	47.28
Comilla	962,696	1,396,973	1,231	1,265	782	1,105	41.30
Noakhali	697,697	784,184	889	879	785	892	13.33
Sylhet	1,003,193	1,269,070	1,431	1,746	701	727	3.71
Dhaka	960,704	1,050,614	1,252	1,151	767	913	19.03
Faridpur	651,508	1,123,820	1,226	1,254	531	896	68.74
Jamalpur	468,405	582,660	640	614	731	949	19.05
Mymensing	1,412,460	1,592,604	1,643	1,541	860	1,033	20.12
Tangil	499,430	556,349	611	634	817	877	7.34
Barisal	735,055	923,043	1,167	1,241	630	744	18.09
Jessore	756,027	1,209,891	1,243	1,208	608	1,002	64.80
Khulna	591,012	712,472	1,032	1,067	573	668	16.58
Kushtia	368,013	634,120	626	628	588	1,010	71.77
Patuakhali	328,718	417,573	639	791	514	528	2.72
Bogra	541,941	836,640	713	706	760	1,185	55.92
Dinajpur	677,604	1,012,351	1,139	1,219	595	784	31.76
Pabna	569,893	648,147	921	819	619	791	27.79
Rajshahi	988,492	1,392,325	1,698	1,706	582	816	40.21
Rangpur	1,281,595	1,658,672	1,687	1,705	760	973	28.03
Bangladesh	14,189,553	18,951,722	20,646	21,246	687	892	29.84

Source: Computed by the author from BBS data

The pattern of food output per acre shows that it is already quite high in the densely populated eastern districts. Hence, further growth is difficult and therefore slow. In the less densely populated western districts, the scope of raising the level of agricultural intensity and other inputs is much greater, and therefore output per acre is growing faster.

Yet another important characteristic of Bangladesh agriculture is that the levels of urbanization and education, which represent social development of a community and are generally believed to have an important influence on agricultural development, are not associated with agricultural growth. Urbanization and educational levels of a community reflect the quality of human capital and have an important influence on agricultural productivity (Evanson and Kisleve 1975, Schultz 1981, Hayami and Ruttan 1985). In turn, agricultural productivity and development open the way for social transformation, which may be reflected in higher levels of urbanization and education. But in Bangladesh, it appears that social organization has lagged behind agricultural development. In other words, agricultural development is not resulting in the social development of the rural community (Dayal 1989). The lack of spatial accord between social development and agricultural productivity has been exhibited for several developing countries (Brown 1971, Antle 1983, Dayal 1984, Kalirajan and Shand 1985). In Bangladesh, the lack of relationship between productivity and education is probably because agriculture is heavily dominated by rice cultivation. Its cultivation is so well established in most areas that there is little scope for improvements in decision making or entrepreneurship. Over a large area the soil is so well adapted for rice that it is now rendered almost unsuitable for other crops (Narain 1965 and Rao 1971). The quality of human capital matters where entrepreneurial decisions can make a difference in production.

Output per agricultural worker

From the point of view of food supply and human welfare, it is perhaps more important to examine changes in food output per agricultural worker. It is an important measure of what farmers get in return for their efforts. Also, an examination of changes in output per worker is important for observing the Malthusian effect of population growth on food supply. However, food output per worker has remained a neglected topic of research in developing countries. Agricultural growth and development has been largely assessed in terms of changes in total production and/or output per unit of land. This approach is commonly taken because labour input is very largely provided by the family members, who are unpaid workers. Therefore, return to land is the main concern. Some believe that the marginal product of labour is zero in subsistence farming, and hence there is not much point in analysing labour productivity.

It is very interesting to note that even in Bangladesh, where the labour force has been continually increasing, the output per worker increased over time. Between 1970-71 and 1991-92, the output of cereals per agricultural worker increased by 28.9 percent. However, if this change is measured from 1972-73, it is only 10.5 percent, or 0.55 percent per year. It is rather disturbing to note that the increase in food output per agricultural worker was very small and far lower than the increase in output per acre. It means that food production in Bangladesh, expectedly, became more labour intensive than it was in the base year. In Bangladesh, output per worker should, theoretically, decline, because the labour force continues to increase without much change in the input of land. But, in reality, the output per agricultural worker has continued to increase, although slowly. Higher intensity of labour leads to higher yields per acre, up to a certain point. Hence, output per worker increases through increased output per unit of land. Dayal (1990) found that output per acre was the most powerful explanatory variable in a regression model to account for changes in output per worker.

Although there are very large differences in food production efficiency per worker across districts, efficiency increased in every district during the period (Table 5.5). High output per worker is found in Chittagong, Chittagong HT, and Noakhali, three densely populated southeastern districts, and also in Jessore, Kushtia, Bogra, and Rajshahi — four less populated western districts, where it was more than 1,400 Takas per worker. An important point to note is that several of the districts that displayed a high level of labour productivity at the end of the reference period also registered high growth rates in output per worker., as for example Chittagong HT, Kushtia, Bogra, and Rajshahi. It seems that special efforts were made in these districts during the reference period to raise productivity. Therefore, labour productivity levels and its growth were both high in the same districts.

Population pressure and agricultural intensification

A heavily populated country like Bangladesh, where the people-land ratio is steadily deteriorating, provides an ideal situation for testing how society, in a densely populated region, responds to further population growth in organizing its food production systems. Boserup (1975) notes that cultivators behave differently in densely populated areas and that it is necessary to examine the effect of population growth in both densely and less densely populated areas.

In recent years, the food output in Bangladesh has increased mainly by increasing the level of agricultural intensity (frequency of cropping). It is, therefore, important to know how rapid population growth is affecting the level of agricultural intensification and, consequently, food output. In this section we examine the relationship between population density and growth on the one hand and agricultural intensity on the other, over time and space in Bangladesh. A positive relationship would suggest that population growth stimulates agricultural growth and a negative relationship would indicate that it is an obstacle to agricultural growth. This relationship has not yet been fully understood, with some scholars believing that it should receive the highest priority in development studies (Robinson and Schutjer 1984). However, the problem has not received much attention in Bangladesh.

This section has two main objectives. The first is to identify the influence of population growth in a densely populated region on agricultural intensity, and hence on output. The second is to examine the influence of regional population density differentials on the spatial dynamics of agricultural intensification, and to present a regional theory of agricultural intensification. The regional theory of agricultural intensification states that agricultural intensity increases in response to population growth, and that therefore at some point in time a strong regional association between agricultural intensity and population density may exist. But high agricultural intensity in the most densely populated regions, after reaching a certain maximum, begins to shift into less densely populated regions in response to continuing national growth of population and demand. Hence, the regional accord between the two variables begins to weaken.

Table 5.5

Regional changes in agricultural labour productivity per male agricultural worker at constant 1969-70 prices

Districts	Value of agricultural production per male agricultural worker		Percentage change in output per worker
	1976-79 avg.	1988-91 avg.	1991 over 1976
Chittagong	1271	1495	17.6
Chittagong HT	901	1655	83.7
Comilla	801	1186	44.7
Noakhali	1334	1423	6.7
Sylhet	923	1108	20.0
Dhaka	887	921	3.8
Faridpur	709	1161	63.7
Jamalpur	931	1099	18.0
Mymensingh	1037	1111	7.1
Tangil	1056	1117	5.8
Barisal	971	1157	19.1
Jessore	979	1488	52.0
Khulna	860	985	14.5
Kushtia	889	1454	63.5
Patuakhali	1122	1351	20.4
Bogra	967	1413	46.6
Dinajpur	981	1390	41.7
Pabna	948	1024	8.0
Rajshahi	1048	1402	33.8
Rangpur	907	1114	22.8
BANGLADESH	951	1206	26.8

Source: Calculated by the author from BBS data

Theoretical considerations

Human concern about the impact of population growth on the quality of life has given rise to the formulation of a number of population theories. The population theory of Thomas Malthus is the most widely known. Drawing on the concept of diminishing returns, Malthus (1798) developed a theory to explain the impact of population growth on human well-being. His main argument was that the growth of resources required to support a population cannot keep pace with the growth of population. He concluded that, while the population grows at a geometric rate, the means of subsistence grow only at an arithmetic rate. Therefore, in a race between food and population, food production inevitably falls behind population growth. Continued growth of population, therefore, leads to hunger, starvation, and absolute poverty.

When Malthus' work was published in 1798, it was highly regarded as an excellent attempt to explain the reality of population growth and its impact on human welfare. In the 19th and 20th centuries, however, his theory began to fall into disfavour due to lack of empirical support, for while European population grew rapidly there also occurred unprecedented increases in living standards. Even today, while Europe is the most densely populated continent of the world, it enjoys very high standards of living. However, one could argue that much of the European prosperity in the 19th and early 20th centuries can be attributed to increasing control of resources outside the continent's geographical boundaries. Several European countries gained control over extensive resources outside Europe by establishing colonies in Asia, Africa, and Latin America. Hence, as population increased the resource base also increased. Europe, therefore, was not a good example to discredit Malthus. More recently, however, Malthus seems to have failed again in Asia, where, in most countries, food production has increased faster than population. Subsistence levels have more than matched increasing population.

Malthusian population theory is now generally regarded as pessimistic, because it completely ignores the positive aspects of population growth on production and technology. The failure of Malthus in Europe, if we ignore colonial benefits, and more recently in Asia, has led to the emergence of several anti-Malthusian models to explain the impact of population growth on human welfare. For example, Clark (1957), Brookfield (1962 and 1972), Boserup (1965, 1975, 1981, 1990) and Simon (1977) are among those who have emphasized the positive contribution of population growth to economic progress. They have argued that population growth creates demand for larger output and thus provides an economic incentive and, perhaps, social obligation to increase production. A subsistence society responds to population growth, first by expansion of cultivated land to increase output, but under rapid population growth such possibilities soon become exhausted. After this stage, direct investment of the rapidly increasing labour supply in labour intensive techniques of production alone can increase output by removing the constraint on output imposed by the shortage of arable land (Boserup 1975, Hossain 1987). Boserup argues that population pressure, rather than being a demographic catastrophe, has been a compelling force for agricultural innovation and for increasing production. She stresses that population growth leads to more intensive methods of production, which in turn necessitate the use of improved technology and practices of production and consequently demand greater input of labour and other inputs (Boserup 1965). "Frequency of cropping is positively related to both population density and technological change." In her later work, she clearly states that increased use of irrigation and fertilizers is a function of population density (Boserup 1981). Thus, Boserup strongly challenges the premise embedded in the classical theory that population growth always leads to a steady decline in labour productivity.

Simon also seems to support the positive impact of population on production. He argues that population growth creates more demand for food and other agricultural products, and thus creates an atmosphere for investment and incentives for increasing output. Under such conditions, any available surplus of labour and capital is invested in the development of new land for agriculture or development of irrigation to permit more intensive use of existing land (Simon 1977, p.253).

Geertz (1963) was struck by the amazing labour-absorbing capacity of wet rice farming in Java. He noticed that wet rice cultivation in Java has absorbed an endless increase in population without any significant drop in individual incomes. This is made possible by an extraordinary ability of wet rice farming to maintain marginal productivity of labour. It implies that an additional input of labour increases total output and output per unit of land and, consequently, maintains labour productivity, although at a low level.

Empirical testing of Boserup's theory

Among those works which have emphasized the positive influence of population growth on output, Boserup's work has became particularly well known. Her thesis that population pressure compels agricultural intensification and innovation and increases production has been tested by several researchers in different environments and at different scales. Brown and Podolefsky (1976) tested the relationship between population density and agricultural intensity in the New Guinea Highlands and found a significant positive correlation between the two. Turner et al. (1977) examined the relationship, using cross-sectional data for one point in time, obtained from 29 tribal communities. They also found a significant positive correlation between population density and agricultural intensity. Further, they pointed out that the correlation strengthens considerably by adding to the model variables representing environmental characteristics such as rainfall. Grossman (1984) examined the relationship over time, using village level data from Samaria, Israel, for three selected years, and found strong support for Boserup.

Pingali and Binswanger (1987) noted that agricultural societies, in general, respond positively to increasing population pressure and market demand. They adopt methods of cultivation and technologies that increase output to meet increased demand. However, there is often some decline in labour productivity, which is not uniform across regions.

There are some commonalities in the above three studies. They have all used cross-sectional data of different quality and scales, and they were all conducted in relatively sparsely populated regions. Hence, they do not give any indication of how a society will respond to population growth over time in organizing its production systems when the population density nearly approaches the extreme end of the spectrum. To answer the above question, Boserup's theory must be tested in the densely populated agrarian regions.

There are several other studies that provide empirical support for Boserup's thesis in low density regions (see for example Clark 1966, Gleve and White 1969, Basehart 1973, Carlstien 1982, Bilsbarrow 1987).

A few studies on this theme also exist for Bangladesh. Chen and Chowdhury (1975), found that in Bangladesh the proportion of land area cropped was positively related to population density. This implies more intensive use of land in densely populated districts.

More recently, the relationship between population pressure and agricultural productivity in Bangladesh was examined by Chaudhury (1981 and 1989), using cross-sectional district data for 1961-64 and 1974-77 averages. He argues that population growth led to a decline in the land-people ratio and consequently to a higher level of multiple cropping and land augmenting inputs per unit area. Despite this he found that the increase in per capita output of foodgrains was insignificant. Boyce (1987) discussed the impact of population growth on agriculture in Bangladesh and found a positive relationship between population growth and growth of per capita output of agriculture for the period between 1949 and 1980, but a negative relationship over a longer period between 1901 and 1980, using cross-sectional and time series data.

All three studies cited above compare pre-1965 subjective data, based on 'eye estimates', with the more accurate data based on crop cutting surveys introduced after 1965. Hence their results could have been affected by comparing data of different quality. The present study differs from the above three in that it uses more recent and reliable data for post independence Bangladesh, and develops a regional theory of agricultural intensity.

A brief review of some studies presented here provides strong support for Boserup. The studies demonstrate that higher population density leads to smaller land area per worker, and consequently to higher intensity of cultivation, higher levels of land augmenting inputs, and increased output per unit area.

The impact of population growth on the depletion of resources has aroused much concern in recent years. Neo-Malthusians argue that increasing population pressure leads to over use of land and consequently to land degradation. This implies that intensive agriculture causes damage to land resources. But this view must be treated with caution, because empirical support for the argument is weak. For example, in several densely populated areas with a long history such as Europe and East Asia there is relatively little damage to land resources. In contrast, in some areas with small populations and a short history there is considerable land degradation (Barrow 1991). Damage to land resources from intensive cultivations can be avoided by suitable measures of land preservation and fertilization (Boserup 1990). Land fertility can be maintained for a long time through careful crop rotation of cereals with legumes, application of organic manure and humus, and minimizing of erosion. However, these sound traits of husbandry are often sacrificed for quick profit (Brookfield et al. 1990). Ehrlich et al. (1977), who are great supporters of Malthus, noted, "Depletion of soil nutrients and humus need not follow from intensive cropping, as demonstrated by the continued fertility of rice fields in Asia that have been cultivated continuously for thousands of years".

The empirical support for Malthus is scanty and largely descriptive because "available quantitative data do not support this theory" (Simon 1981). Writers who support Malthusian ideas argue that more people use more resources and cause a general deterioration of natural and social environments and create scarcity (Overbeek 1976, Eckholm 1976, Ehrlich 1968, Coale and Hoover 1958, Meadows et al. 1972). Meadows et al. (1992), twenty years after the publication of *The Limits To Growth*, have revised their previous stand and sound more optimistic. Some researchers have maintained that degradation of resources and environment is more due to rapidly increasing consumption standards and cost-saving quick technology than population growth (Brookfield 1990, Butzar 1990). "Often enough relatively small populations have done great damage to the environment — sometimes to the point where a way of life has had to be given up, allowing the ecosystem to recuperate, while the remaining human population is forced to reevaluate and re-formulate its priorities and strategies" (Butzar 1990).

Perhaps it is right to say that Malthus has proven wrong but the Malthusian concern persists (Turner and Kate 1990, p.14).

Population growth

From very early times, agricultural development in Bangladesh has taken place against a backdrop of rapid population growth. British political control over Bengal created demand for several agricultural commodities and encouraged the expansion of agriculture in under-utilized regions. The industrial revolution in Europe, and the consequent growth of industries and population, created large demands for food and agricultural raw materials. These developments in Europe had important implications for agricultural growth in Bengal. As rural population growth was not accompanied by a parallel growth in the manufacturing sector, it must have led to an increase in population pressure on agricultural land. Blyn (1966, p.135) reported that the population density in Bengal around the middle of the 18th century was twice as high as in Punjab. During a fifty year period (1881 to 1931), the population of Bengal doubled, reaching an average density of 1,000 persons per square mile or 391 per sq. km (Blyn 1966). Geddes (1937) attributed the rapid growth of population in Bangladesh (former Greater Bengal) to the natural ecology, which is similar to that of several other very densely populated regions in Asia such as Kerala in India and Java in Indonesia.

Continued growth of population pressure led to the expansion of agricultural land throughout the 18th and 19th centuries. In some parts of Bengal, the expansion of agricultural land had already reached its physical limits by the end of the 19th century, and even the most marginal land was used to produce cheap inferior food for the poor (Kelly 1981). When opportunities for the expansion of cultivation on new land became exhausted, rapidly increasing population pressure led to increased intensity of cultivation on existing land. This is evidenced by the extent of the net cropped area, which has remained almost unchanged from the middle of the present century although total area under foodgrain increased considerably (Figure 1). There is also evidence that application of manure on rice crops began as early as the 1870s (Kelly 1981).

Time series data compiled by Islam (1978) for Dacca and Chittagong divisions also clearly indicate that the net cropped area (a good proxy for cultivated land) remained almost unchanged between 1920 and 1945. In Greater Bengal, the cultivated area generally declined during the same period (Blyn 1966). Chaudhury (1989) reports continuation of the trend to the present. Although this decline in cultivated area may sound puzzling, it is real, and could be due to a combination of several factors. As population grew rapidly some land might have become marginal due to over-use and therefore abandoned, while some was taken up by expanding settlements and lateral shifting of river channels (Haque and Hossain 1988). Hence there is good documentary evidence that while the population of Bangladesh has continued to increase rapidly, the net cultivated area has not.

The inter-censal growth rates were quite erratic up to the 1951 census, but thereafter they began to increase quite rapidly (Table 5.6). The population more than doubled between 1951 and 1991. It increased from 44 million to almost 110 million during the period. However, since 1974 there appears to be some decline in the growth rates. It seems that population growth in Bangladesh peaked in the early 1970s and thereafter it began to decline (Table 5.6). The decline in the growth rates of population is due to an increase in family planning activities. For example, the use of condoms between 1971 and 1991 increased by more than six times. It is comforting to note that at long last the idea of population control is being accepted by the people.

The average population density of Bangladesh at present stands at 1,600 persons per square mile (625 per sq. km), an extremely high density indeed for an agrarian economy. The density figures for the total area do not show the full reality. The gravity of the excessive population problem is exposed when one considers density on net cropped area, which was 4.1 persons per acre in 1991, far greater than densities found in China, India, Japan, and Indonesia. In some *thanas* of Bangladesh, population density on net cropped area is as high as 11.3 people per acre. Such high density has produced an extremely high people-land ratio in Bangladesh, which is worsening. Bangladesh is now one of the few countries in Asia where population is still growing at the annual rate of more than 2.0 percent. Tabah (1982) predicts that population density on the total area in Bangladesh in the year 2025 will be five times the current density of Japan.

Over a very large area, from Comilla in the southeast to Rangpur in the northwest, the population density is more than 650 persons per square kilometre. The coastal districts and Chittagong HT are less densely populated, and generally

Table 5.6
Population growth in Bangladesh

Census years	Population in millions	Exponential growth rates
1901	28.9	-
1911	31.5	0.94
1921	33.2	0.60
1931	35.6	0.74
1941	42.0	1.70
1951	44.1	0.50
1961	55.2	2.26
1974	76.4	2.48
1981	89.9	2.35
1991	109.9	2.03

Source: *Statistical Yearbok of Bangladesh 1992*

have densities below 350 persons per square kilometres. The remaining districts, namely Sylhet, Dinajpur, parts of Rajshahi, Kushtia, and Jessore, have intermediate densities.

The regional pattern of population growth indicates that population is growing faster then the national average in Tangil and Dhaka, which are already densely populated districts. In the western region, above average growth of population between 1974 and 1991 was recorded in Bogra, Dinajpur, Pabna, and Rajshahi. In these four districts the pressure of population on cultivated land is well below the national average, and therefore they offer better scope for absorption of additional population in the agricultural sector (Tables 5.7 and 5.10).

Despite the declining land resources per capita, Bangladesh manages to feed its population largely from its own production, as less than 8 percent of the food requirements are imported or received in aid. A cursory inspection of average yield data of major food crops suggests that they are not high even by Asian standards. Hence, the only conclusion one can draw is that Bangladesh is able to feed about 90 percent of its large population by maximizing total output per unit of existing land through increasing yield per acre and multiple cropping.

Continued population growth has produced a great deal of landlessness and a large number of small but productive and intensively cultivated agricultural holdings. It has been noted previously that output per unit of land (land productivity) is relatively high in densely populated regions, where agricultural holdings are small. This relationship appears to be initiated by increases in

Table 5.7
Regional pattern of rural population growth

Districts	Population 1974 (000)	Population 1991 (000)	Percentage change
Chittagong HT	456	528	15.79
Chittagong	3410	4578	34.25
Comilla	5572	7520	34.96
Noakhali	3165	4122	30.24
Sylhet	4628	6099	31.78
Dhaka	5361	8088	64.20
Faridpur	3943	5053	22.45
Mymensingh	7143	9712	35.96
Tangil	1969	2720	38.14
Barisal	3774	4727	25.25
Jessore	3146	4284	36.17
Khulna	3037	3885	27.92
Kushtia	1727	2352	36.19
Patuakhali	1462	1833	25.38
Bogra	2148	3064	42.18
Dinajpur	2458	3526	43.45
Pabna	2600	3626	39.46
Rajshahi	4021	5726	42.40
Rangpur	5185	6925	33.56
Bangladesh	65,205	88,946	36.41

Source: Computed by the authors from the BBS data

population pressure on land resources. If the scope for the expansion of cultivated land is very limited, an increase in population pressure leads to a more intensive use of land and, consequently, to higher output per unit of land. In such a situation, because land becomes a scarce and therefore expensive factor of production, producers prefer to use more of other inputs on a fixed amount of land. They try to maximize returns to land. There is good deal of evidence that this is happening in Bangladesh (Chaudhury 1981).

Relationship between population density and agricultural intensity in Bangladesh

I examined the relationship between population density and agricultural intensity using time series and cross-sectional data. Agricultural intensity is the dependent variable and is defined as the ratio of net cropped are to total cropped area. This measures frequency of cultivation, a measure of agricultural intensity also used by Boserup. National time series data, cross-sectional district data for agricultural intensity, and population data were all obtained from various issues of the *Statistical Yearbook of Bangladesh* (Government of Bangladesh 1982, 1984, 1988, 1993). Time series were deliberately not extended further back because before 1965 acreage data were not fully reliable.

Agricultural intensity as defined here includes neither the levels of inputs used nor the methods of cultivation, but it does imply that a higher frequency of cultivation will require higher inputs of labour and possibly other inputs.

Agricultural intensity in a given area may be affected by a variety of variables such as population pressure on land resources, quality of environment, farm size and the extent of its fragmentation, land tenure systems, availability and cost of irrigation and other yield augmenting inputs, market price of output, accessibility to markets, and the political economy of the region. But some of these variables are unquantifiable and they exert only an indirect influence on agricultural intensity. The data on most of the other variables in the list are often not available in developing countries over a desired span of time or spatial scale. Where available, the data on the consumption of inputs, particularly inputs of unpaid labour, are less reliable than data on land use. The most satisfactory measure of agricultural intensity would be the value of all agricultural inputs per unit of land. However, the data required for such an index can be obtained only through intensive fieldwork. In developing countries, like Bangladesh, this would mean careful monitoring of farmers' activities throughout the year, because most farmers do not keep a complete record of the inputs used, particularly the input of their own labour. Even if it were possible to do this rigorous exercise, it would provide a measurement of agricultural intensity only for one year and for a small area. For this reason, Boserup's thesis cannot be quantitatively examined at the village level in Bangladesh and for the same reason in any developing country. Therefore, when the objective is to analyse changes over time and space at a macro scale, one has to depend on types of secondary data on selected variables that may sound most satisfactory. Hence, several researchers have employed partial measures of agricultural intensity based on some selected variables. For example, Dayal (1974) measured agricultural intensity in terms of stocking density in a dairy farming region; Eder (1977) measured it in terms of a shift from rice to vegetable cultivation; Grossman (1984) measured it in terms of a shift from grain to olive cultivation in Samaria. Subramaniyan and Nirmala (1991) measured intensity in terms of gross area sown per capita. Turner et al. (1977), Chaudhury (1981), Pingali and Binswanger (1987), and Chaudhary and Anjea (1991) all measured agricultural intensity in terms of frequency of cropping.

It seems that an index based on more frequent use of land is a simple and therefore the most widely used indicator of agricultural intensity. It is based on land use data which are generally more reliable and available for longer spans of time thus permitting construction of time series. Boserup (1965) measured agricultural intensity in terms of frequency of cultivation in traditional agriculture. She explained that population growth creates greater demand for agricultural output and at the same time leads to sub-division and fragmentation of agricultural holdings. This is particularly true for Bangladesh agriculture (Chaudhury 1989). Farms become smaller in size but are required to produce more. Farmers, therefore, begin to use land more intensively in order to maximize output. Initially, they may increase the input of their own labour, but they soon realize that as agricultural land is cultivated more frequently the use of other yield-augmenting inputs becomes imperative in order to prevent productivity decline. Boserup (1965) stated, " There is thus a close association between the system of fallow and the techniques of fertilization". There is strong empirical support for a positive association between frequency of cultivation on the one hand, and greater use of labour, fertilizers, and irrigation on the other (Singh 1975, Dayal 1977, Pingali and Binswanger 1987, Subramaniyan and Nirmala 1991 to mention only a few). Khan (1985) found that agricultural intensity in terms of frequency of cultivation accounts for more than half the increase in labour input. Hence, it is assumed that frequency of cultivation adequately incorporates the use of other inputs besides labour.

Rural population density was computed over net cropped area. This measure provides nutritional density for each region and is the most appropriate indicator of population pressure on land resources. Time series for rural population density were derived from population census data, using interpolation and extrapolation techniques and inter-census growth rates.

Boserup's theory of agricultural intensification is a demand theme theory of agricultural change (Turner 1989). It emphasizes that agricultural growth is in response to increases in demand for agricultural output, particularly food. The demand, in turn, is determined by the total population. Even in primitive societies, some members of the community are engaged in non-agricultural activities, but they too contribute to the demand for agricultural output.

Agriculture in Bangladesh, like that of most other Asian countries, is no longer entirely subsistence oriented. National and regional market demands have had an important influence on the land use systems. Cultivators and landowners both have market incentives for producing a surplus. Because Bangladesh is a food deficit country, any surplus can be readily sold in the market. It is common knowledge that even subsistence farmers must sell part of the output in the market in order to have some cash income for buying things that they cannot produce. In Bangladesh 75 percent of the paddy farmers sell part of their produce for cash income (Quasem 1987). The size of the surplus that cultivators and landowners aim to produce depends on the prevailing market prices, which, in turn, are determined by the demand created by both the rural and urban populations at the regional and national levels. Nevertheless, in a predominantly agrarian society, a great bulk of the demand is determined by the rural population. Further, the essential pre-condition for agricultural intensification is the increase in rural population, which provides additional labour for more frequent cultivation of land (Boserup 1965, p.95). The rural population density, therefore, has a more direct influence on agricultural intensity.

Further, Bangladesh is one of the least urbanized countries of the world (Khan 1982). Therefore there are very high correlations between the growth rates and distribution patterns of total and rural populations ($r=0.99$ for growth rates, based on Khan 1982; and $r=0.98$ for distribution, calculated by the author). There is, therefore, little difference in the distribution patterns and growth rates of total and rural population. Hence, the rural population strongly represents growth and distributional characteristics of the total population, and adequately represents national demand for food and other agricultural commodities.

First, using time series data for the period 1965 to 1991, I examined the relationship between agricultural intensity and rural population density on net cropped area, which is a good approximation of cultivated land in Bangladesh. Second, using cross-sectional district data, I examined the regional association between the two variables for 1974 and 1991, two population census years. I selected 1974 because it was the first population census year for independent Bangladesh and very close to 1972-73, the base year in this study, and 1991 was the latest census year. The rural population densities for the population census years were expected to be more accurate than densities for inter-censal years. Third, I examined the regional association between the growth of the two variables between 1974 and 1991. I could not use a more refined spatial scale because agricultural land use data for areal units smaller than a district were not available after 1982-83. Since agricultural intensity is subject to annual fluctuations, I used three-year averages, i.e., the 1971-74 average and the 1988-91 average.

Results and Discussion

Largely based on the documentary evidence in an earlier section of this chapter, it was argued that population density in Bangladesh has been increasing over a long time and that there has been no noticeable change in the net cropped area. This implies that most of the increase in agricultural output has been through intensification of agriculture. In this section the relationship between agricultural intensity and population density will be more objectively determined.

Agricultural intensity in Bangladesh is subject to annual fluctuations because it is affected by weather conditions and natural disasters, particularly rainfall, floods, and cyclones. It often drops below the average trend in bad years but rises again in favourable years. Therefore, the intensity index cannot move only in one direction. However, the over all trend would show the direction of change. Between 1965 and 1991, the agricultural intensity in Bangladesh displayed an unmistakably strong

Table 5.8

Relationship between rural population density and agricultural intensity over time, 1965 to 1991

Years	Rural population density on NCA	Agricultural intensity NCA/TCA*100
1964-65	2.53	135
1965-66	2.53	137
1966-67	2.65	137
1967-68	2.64	144
1968-69	2.71	143
1969-70	2.75	151
1970-71	2.87	142
1971-72	3.07	138
1972-73	3.07	139
1973-74	3.11	140
1974-75	3.23	139
1975-76	3.23	141
1976-77	3.37	142
1977-78	3.39	143
1978-79	3.48	153
1979-80	3.48	153
1980-81	3.49	154
1981-82	3.55	154
1982-83	3.60	155
1983-84	3.66	154
1984-85	3.74	152
1985-86	3.76	154
1986-87	3.79	151
1987-88	4.12	155
1988-89	4.26	161
1989-90	4.24	162
1990-91	4.40	172

Correlation between agricultural intensity and time

R^2= 0.745, F= 73.048, N= 27,   Significant at >.001 level

Correlation between agricultural intensity and rural population density over time

R^2= 0.734, F=68.942, N= 27,   Significant at > .001 level

Source: Calculated by the author from BBS data

positive trend, which is confirmed by the positive correlation and regression

117

positive trend, which is confirmed by the positive correlation and regression coefficients (Table 5.8). During the 20 year period, the positive trend of agricultural intensity was interrupted twice (Figure 5.1). The first interruption was in the early 1970s, when it dropped substantially. This represented partial dislocation of agriculture caused by the war of liberation followed by a series of serious natural disasters - floods, cyclones, and hailstones-some of which were the worst in living memory. However, agriculture made a remarkable recovery by the end of 1970s. The second interruption, in the early 1980s, represents devastating floods in 1980, droughts in 1981 and 1982, and again serious floods in 1984. But from 1978 onward agricultural intensity continued to rise, despite natural disasters, (Table 5.8 and Figure 5.1). The coefficients are highly significant at the .001 level when agricultural intensity is regressed against time and also rural population density.

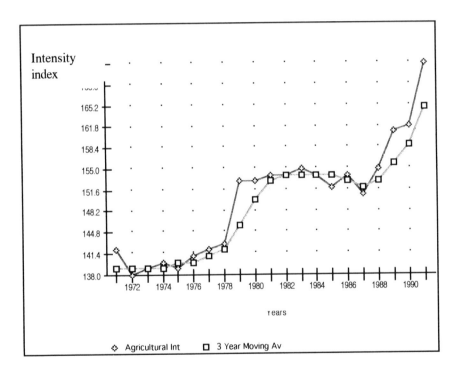

Figure 5.1 Agricultural intensity over time

It appears that the rising rural population pressure on cultivated land was the main force behind the growth of agricultural intensity over time. This is confirmed by a positive correlation between rural population density and agricultural

Table 5.9
Regional relationship between rural population density and agricultural intensity,1974

Distrcts	Rural population density on NCA 1974	Agricultural intensity NCA/TCA*100 1971-74
Chittagong HT	2.64	158
Chittagong	4.32	136
Comilla	4.32	155
Noakhali	3.42	147
Sylhet	2.66	125
Dhaka	4.28	145
Faridpur	3.31	158
Mymensingh	2.92	167
Tangil	3.45	157
Barisal	3.21	146
Jessore	2.54	125
Khulna	3.10	115
Kushtia	2.84	120
Patuakhali	2.28	125
Bogra	3.02	149
Dinajpur	2.20	129
Pabna	3.29	146
Rajshahi	2.44	125
Rangpur	3.12	177
Bangladesh	3.11	144

Variables	**Regression Results**		
	Simple correlation coefficient	Regression coefficient	t statistics
Agricultural intensity (Dependent variable)	-	-	-
Rural population density on NCA	0.77	29.49	5.08[b]
Constant	-	47.88	2.66[a]
R^2=0.59, N=19, F=25.9			

a Significant at .01 level
b Significant at >.001 level
Source: Calculated by the author from BBS data

intensity, which is statistically highly significant (Table 5.8). The growth of agricultural intensity might have been helped by the expansion of irrigation and HYVs, but the motive force was population growth and the consequent rise in demand for food. After having established a strong positive relationship between agricultural intensity and population pressure on agricultural land over time at the national scale, it is assumed that such an association must also exist across regions for the same causal mechanism. It is important to note that the spatial accord between rural population density on net cropped area and agricultural intensity appears to be weakening over time. In 1974, the regional association between the two variables was quite strong. The rural population density on cultivated land accounted for about 60 percent of the regional variation in agricultural intensity (Table 5.9). However, in 1991 the association had become very weak, though still statistically significant. In 1991, the rural population density accounted for only 20 percent of the regional variation in agricultural intensity (Table 5.10). The weakening of the geographical association between the two variables over time gives a hint that the regional growth pattern of agricultural intensity is undergoing a change. Therefore, I examined the regional relationship between the growth rates of the two variables across districts, during 1974 and 1991. The results confirmed the suspicion that agricultural intensity is no longer continuing to increase only in the densely populated regions in response to increasing population pressure. Agricultural intensity was beginning to rise even in the less populated districts. It may be noted that in 1991, the highest levels of agricultural intensity were found in some less densely populated districts, namely Rangpur, Bogra, and Mymensingh (Table 5.10). There was practically no regional association between the growth rates of the two variables (Table 5.11).

The regional association between the two variables in 1974, although positive and highly significant, was clearly not as strong as the association over time at the national scale. This indicates a definite change in the growth patterns of the two variables.

Regression analysis reveals a strong positive relationship between agricultural intensity and derived rural population densities over time. But the regional association between agricultural intensity and rural population density is weakening. The lack of regional accord in the growth rates of the two variables suggests that population growth can no longer lead to further intensification of agriculture in some areas. It could be that the intensification of agricultural production, through multiple cropping, has already reached saturation in some of the densely populated areas. The weak existing regional accord in the distribution of the two variables may be a legacy of the past, when agricultural intensification responded positively to population growth even in the relatively densely populated regions. The indications now are that this accord may be completely obliterated in the near future, as intensification of agriculture now appears to be taking place in less densely populated regions.

Table 5.10

Regional relationship between rural population density and agricultural intensity — 1991

Districts	Rural population density on NCA 1991	Agricultural intensity NCA/TCA* 1988-91
Chittagong HT	2.89	143
Chittagong	6.34	166
Cimilla	5.92	178
Noakhali	4.69	163
Sylhet	3.73	145
Dhaka	6.42	166
Faridpur	4.25	169
Mymensingh	3.97	180
Tangil	4.46	173
Barisal	3.90	148
Jessore	3.54	155
Khulna	3.62	131
Kushtia	3.72	163
Patuakhali	2.47	143
Bogra	4.22	191
Dinajpur	2.80	148
Pabna	3.75	174
Rajshahi	3.33	134
Rangpur	4.04	191
Bangladesh	4.16	162

Regression Results

Variables	Simple correlation coefficient	Regression coefficient	t Statistics
Agricultural intensity (Dependent Variable)	-	-	-
Rural population density on NCA	0.455	7.814	2.166[a]
Constant	-	130.324	8.528[b]

R^2=0.207, N =19, F =4.69

a   Significant at > .05 level
b   "   > .001
Source: Calculated by the author from BBS data

121

Hence, the results of this study open up some interesting points for debate. Perhaps the relationship between population pressure and agricultural intensity is not consistent over space. Perhaps it depends on regional conditions relating to environmental quality and the population-resource ratio and not on population pressure alone (Brown and Podolefsky 1976).

A strong positive regional association between agricultural intensity and population density has been found, so far, only in some sparsely populated regions (Brown and Podolefsky 1976, Turner et al 1977, Grossman 1984, Pingali and Biswanger 1987). Bangladesh exhibits an entirely different situation from the situations presented in the above studies. In their samples, an increase in population led to an increase in intensity because of the possibility of tapping existing unrealized potential. By contrast, in the densely populated regions of Bangladesh, there is perhaps no unrealized potential for increasing the frequency of cultivation. Population pressure has already compelled farmers to raise the frequency of cultivation to its maximum level. So an important question arises, i.e., how do people respond to increased population size and consequent increase in labour supply in rural areas where intensification of agriculture may be near the maximum level? Perhaps Boserup had this question in mind while developing her theory. She, therefore, stresses the point that each stage of agricultural intensification will also involve some change in technology. In a situation where increasing the frequency of cultivation is no longer feasible, increased labour supply will be used for more elaborate preparation of fields and implementation of improved but labour-intensive technology such as irrigation of crops, application of manure, use of better implements. This will promote an increase in the output per unit area without any increase in the frequency of cultivation.

It appears that the changes in agricultural intensity, in response to population growth, pass through two distinct stages. During the first stage, intensity increases through multiple cropping, which of course requires an increase in the use of several inputs, but that option is exhausted after some time. During the second stage, the intensity increases only through greater use of inputs per unit of land, without any change in the frequency of cultivation. Among these two stages, the first is relatively cheaper as it does not involve much investment in purchased inputs.

In the densely populated districts of Bangladesh, we encounter a situation where further increases in population cannot lead to a higher frequency of cultivation because it is already at its maximum. In Bangladesh, this level appears to be when the index of agricultural intensity exceeds 170, or when more than 70 percent of the NCA is cropped more than once. (The percentage of NCA used for multiple cropping is always less than 100 because some area is always required for fallow, permanent tree crops, and other long duration crops such as sugar cane.) In Bangladesh, the areas where the intensity index is over 170, such as the north-central and some southeastern districts, may now be in the second stage of intensification. Compared with the level of inputs used in Japanese and West

Table 5.11
Percentage change in rural population density and agricultural intensity across districts between 1974 and 1991

Districts	Rural population density % change	Agricultural intensity % change
Chittagong HT	7.58	-9.49
Chittagong	46.76	22.06
Comilla	37.04	14.84
Noakhali	37.13	10.88
Sylhet	40.22	16.00
Dhaka	50.35	14.48
Faridpur	32.81	6.96
Mymensingh	27.54	9.58
Tangil	27.43	10.19
Barisal	21.49	1.37
Jessore	39.37	24.00
Khulna	16.77	13.91
Kushtia	31.45	35.83
Patuakhali	8.33	14.40
Borga	37.46	28.19
Dinajpur	27.27	14.73
Pabna	20.06	19.18
Rajshahi	36.47	7.20
Rangpur	29.49	7.91
Bangladesh	36.39	12.50

Regression results

Variables	Simple correlation coefficient	Regression coefficient	t Statistics
Agricultural intensity (Dependent variable)	-	-	-
Rural population density	0.442	0.189	0.979*
Constant		9.145	1.432*
$R^2 = 0.195$, N=19, F=4.117			

* Not significant

Source: Calculated by the author from BBS data

European agriculture, it appears that Bangladesh still has plenty of scope for the latter option, limited only by the purchasing power of the farmers. During the second stage, a positive association between population density and land productivity is more likely.

A regional theory of agricultural intensity

In response to population growth, the frequency of cultivation cannot continue to increase indefinitely in a given area. As a result, the spatial concentration of high frequency of cropping appears to shift from high to low population density regions over time. Consider, for example, a country X, divided into three regions, A, B, and C, and suppose that the general quality of land in region A is better than in regions B and C. Given these circumstances, region A will be more conducive to intensive agriculture and will have a higher carrying capacity. It will become more densely populated, relative to other regions, because it will produce a given quantity of output at a lower cost. In contrast, regions B and C being less productive will be initially less populated. The change from less intensive to more intensive agriculture will follow a similar sequence. An increase in population pressure in region A may first lead to a higher level of frequency of cultivation there, but after some time the highest possible limit of the frequency of cultivation may be reached in this region. A further increase of population in region A will undoubtedly create more demand and higher food prices in region A and also at the national level. At this point, farmers in region A, being motivated by higher prices, will be encouraged to pass into the more expensive second stage of agricultural intensification, i.e., using more labour and purchased inputs per unit of land in order to produce more without any change in the frequency of cultivation. Since it is no longer possible to increase the frequency of cultivation in region A, producers in regions B and C will take advantage of A's increased demand and prices. They will begin to increase production through the relatively cheaper first stage of agricultural intensification. This assumes inter-regional mobility of agricultural output.

In fact, inter-regional movement of foodgrains in Bangladesh has increased considerably due to the expansion of transport and communication and withdrawal of several restrictions that were previously part of government policy. Also, the government procurement program, in a way, encourages inter-regional mobility because procurements in one region are often sold in other regions according to need. Therefore, several recent studies on price responsiveness of agricultural output have found that it is on the increase in Bangladesh (Rehman 1987, Alam 1992). Hence, motivated by demand the frequency of cultivation will begin to increase in regions B and C, and may ultimately reach levels as high as in region A (Figure 5.2). An increase in intensification of agriculture will create additional demand for labour and may initiate some migration from region A to regions B and C.

Whether that is actually happening is hard to say in the absence of proper internal migration data. The Bangladesh Population Census gives only decadal net gain or loss of life-time migrants in a district, which is not quite suitable for drawing conclusions about internal movements of population. Nevertheless, regional population growth and fertility data do give some indication of population movements from southeastern and central districts to the western districts. The annual growth rates of population are much higher in the western districts compared with the southeastern and central (Table 5.12). The large differences in the growth rates between the two groups of districts cannot be due to differences in the natural increase, because the fertility rates are about the same, except for Tangil. Hence, the data presented in Table 5.12 does give some indication of net immigration in the western districts between 1971 and 1981.

COUNTRY - X

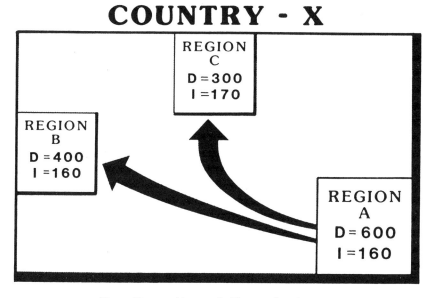

D = Density of Population
I = Intensity of Cultivation

Figure 5.2   Regional shifts in agricultural intensity

However, for a long time population density in region A will remain higher than in regions B and C, because it may depend on several factors such as relative location, land productivity, historical events, and pattern of landownership. High population densities in region A will have become deeply rooted in the local environment and will have produced an inertia that lingers.

Higher frequency of cropping in regions B and C may involve higher costs because a higher level of inputs will be required, e.g. irrigation, fertilizers, and relatively more expensive labour. Therefore, multiple cropping in regions B and C will commence only when food prices are sufficiently high to cover extra costs. It appears that poor environmental conditions tend to lower the level of agricultural intensity until it is economically and socially worthwhile to develop and use technology to overcome the environmental constraints. The explanation for the logical sequence of change from low to high agricultural intensity in country X will be similar to Ricardo's explanation of land rent (Barlowe 1972, Ricardo 1987). In those sparsely populated regions, where environmental conditions for high agricultural intensity are less favourable, increased demand and higher prices in the national market may provide incentive for investments in irrigation and other yield-augmenting inputs and lead to higher levels of agricultural intensity. This will

Table 5.12
Population density, growth rates, fertility, and cropping intensity in selected districts

Districts	Density per square mile of total area	Population growth rates (annual)	Fertility children<4 yrs per female of age 15-49	Cropping intensity (TCA/NSA)*100
Southeastern and central districts				
Comilla	2701	1.70	0.831	169
Noakhali	1810	1.23	0.832	152
Chittagong	1907	1.43	0.796	158
Mymensingh	1863	1.00	0.810	198
Tangil	2123	1.98	0.748	171
Western districts				
Rajshahi	1443	2.35	0.841	132
Dinajpur	1262	2.50	0.829	132
Bogra	1817	2.22	0.797	176
Jessore	1584	2.04	0.860	138
Kushtia	1726	2.11	0.860	138

Source: Calculated by the author from BBS data

break the similarities in the distribution patterns of population density and frequency of cultivation. Bangladesh appears to be at that stage of the agricultural intensity cycle. One gets no significant association between population density and frequency of cultivation if one uses cross-sectional data for growth rates, indicating that agricultural intensity is not responding to population growth any more in some areas.

There appears to be considerable empirical evidence to support the above theory in Bangladesh. For example, in 1974 the highest agricultural intensity index of more than 170 was found only in one district, Rangpur. In 1991, intensity index values of more than 170 were found in six districts and were mainly concentrated in the relatively sparsely populated western districts (Table 5.10). There is considerable evidence to show that a high frequency of cropping, over the past 20 years or so, has moved from the densely populated districts to the relatively less densely populated districts in Bangladesh. It appears that in the more densely populated regions, in the southeast, further increase in population may lead to a higher application of labour and other inputs per unit of land in cultivation, but increasing the frequency of cultivation may no longer be feasible.

The shift of high agricultural intensity, if measured in terms of frequency of cultivation, from more densely populated regions to relatively less densely populated regions in Bangladesh is unique and presents an interesting base for a re-examination of Boserup's model. Boserup (1965) argues that rural population increases will promote a direct investment of labour in agriculture that will expand cultivators' productive capacity. Additional labour supply, as a result of rural population growth, may be used in agriculture in three different ways: 1) for bringing new land under cultivation; 2) for more frequent cultivation of existing land; 3) for the application of improved but labour-intensive technology in cultivation. In Bangladesh, the first option has been almost exhausted everywhere and the second has also been practically exhausted in the densely populated central and southeastern regions. This is clearly exhibited by a declining regional correlation between the two variables. Therefore, high agricultural intensity is not found only in the densely populated regions but it has flowed over into relatively less populated regions as well. Booth (1988) also found a similar situation in Java.

The above analysis directs attention to an important point that has not been debated by Boserup, i.e., the limitations of increasing agricultural intensity. Obviously, one cannot expect cultivation intensity to keep rising indefinitely. Each of the three options, stated earlier, in response to population growth has its limitations. The first will come to an end when there is no more land left within the national boundaries for the expansion of agricultural production. If some land is still available its development may be beyond the economic and technological capabilities of the nation. The second option (increasing the frequency of cultivation) will come to an end when:

$$\sum_{i=1}^{n} DCi = 365 - (\sum_{i=1}^{n} Ti + K) \text{ ------------ } (1)$$

where DCi represents the duration of crop i, and Ti the time between harvesting of crop i and the sowing of the next, and K is the minimum area required for fallow and tree crops. This simply means that land is occupied by some crops almost throughout the year. Hence any increase in demand cannot increase frequency of cropping any further. The second option will end when there is no more land and time to produce an additional crop, a situation described in equation (1). The third option will come to an end when the average output per worker is less than the amount required for subsistence, or when additional output is less than the cost of purchased inputs used in its production. When the first two options are exhausted, further intensification of agricultural production is achieved by increasing the level of inputs per unit of land, which is expensive. Therefore, long before the third option is exhausted in the densely populated regions of a nation, high agricultural intensity begins to flow over into less densely populated regions. Hence, at a given point in time, high agricultural intensity may occur in densely and less densely populated regions at the same time. Bangladesh, at present, appears to be at this stage of agricultural intensification. There is a strong positive relationship between population density and agricultural intensity over time, a modest positive relationship across regions, but no regional accord in the growth rates of the two variables.

Summary and conclusion

Increases in agricultural intensity in a given region may be attributed to various causes but demand created by rapidly growing population appears to be the most important. This study, therefore, examined the relationship between population density and agricultural intensity in Bangladesh, using both time series and cross-sectional data. The results of this analysis strongly support Boserup's thesis and provide an extension of her theory. They also tie in well with the results of the studies reviewed earlier.

There is unmistakable evidence that agricultural intensity has consistently increased in Bangladesh over time along with rapidly growing population and has contributed to increases in agricultural output. There is also a modest but positive relationship between the regional distributions of agricultural intensity and population density. But there is no regional accord in the annual average growth rates of the two variables. These results open up some interesting points for debate, and encourage the development of a regional theory of population growth and agricultural intensity. It is obvious that the frequency of cultivation cannot go on increasing indefinitely in densely populated regions. It was noted that agricultural intensity had already reached a near maximum level in some densely populated regions and was not responding much to further population growth. In order to explain the above situation, I have developed a regional theory of agricultural intensification. The theory states that in the densely populated regions, agricultural intensity, if measured in terms of frequency of cultivation, after reaching a certain maximum level ceases to respond positively to further growth of population and demand. After this point, motivated by market forces, it begins to flow over into less densely populated regions. Hence, the established regional association between population density and agricultural intensity begins to weaken.

It appears that in Bangladesh the levels of agricultural intensity in the densely populated central and southeastern regions have now reached saturation point, if intensity is measured in terms of frequency of cultivation. In these regions, a high level of agricultural intensity is, perhaps, maintained by using more inputs of labour and capital per unit of land, because increasing the frequency of cultivation any further is probably not practical. In the relatively sparsely populated western and northwestern regions, on the other hand, a high level of agricultural intensity is attained by raising the frequency of cultivation.

It is very likely that the regional theory of agricultural intensification presented in this paper may also apply to other Third World countries which do not produce much agricultural surplus for export and where production is largely determined by national demand.

Since there is not much scope for further expansion of agricultural land in Bangladesh, additional agricultural output for the increasing population must come from more frequent use of land or increasing crop yields. But increasing crop yields is a more expensive alternative. Further, more intensive use of land is not only relatively cheap, it also absorbs more labour and thereby helps in lowering unemployment in a labour surplus agrarian economy. Therefore, promotion of intensive agriculture and the monitoring of its shifts over space and time must be an important part of government agricultural development policy. The results of this study may provide a useful guide for agricultural development policy.

Although there is considerable scope for further intensification of agriculture in Bangladesh, it is not the same everywhere. It would, therefore, be more effective if the limited resources were to be used to promote intensive agriculture where conditions appear to be more promising. For example, a policy to encourage more frequent use of land will be more successful in the western and northwestern districts. Here the government policy should be to offer attractive prices for the output and allow its free movement in order to maximize production. This should not raise any serious problems because the government already intervenes in the foodgrain markets through the Foodgrain Procurement Program and the Public Food Distribution System.

The scope for increasing agricultural intensity has increased enormously because of the introduction and rapid spread of fertilizer use in Bangladesh. In this area, the government can encourage further intensification of agriculture by providing fertilizers at subsidized rates to small farmers, particularly in the southeastern districts where the scope for increasing the frequency of cultivation is very limited. Even international aid organizations can channel some of the aid in the form of fertilizers for small farmers. It is important to bring fertilizers within easy reach of small farmers.

The agricultural intensity trend over time in response to population growth and its shifts over space suggest that there is still considerable scope for increasing agricultural output in Bangladesh, despite a very low land-people ratio. As population control programs are already under way, it is possible that even Bangladesh may be able to escape the Malthusian trap.

6 Food consumption patterns

Introduction

Food is essential for the physiological, social, and emotional needs of the people. Although it is necessary for all people, the quantity and quality of food consumed are determined by a complex set of factors. These factors are derived from the earliest phases of the history of the people and are influenced by the geographic, economic, social, and cultural environments. The type of food consumed by the people is deeply embedded in their culture. It is beyond the scope of this chapter to provide the depth of understanding of the complex processes that determine the pattern of food consumption in Bangladesh. The objective of the contents of this chapter is to provide some understanding of the factors that have influenced food consumption patterns in Bangladesh.

Factors affecting quantity and quality of food intake

The food consumption pattern in a region is influenced by a number of interrelated factors, such as land capability, history, social and cultural background, level of economic and technological development, trading links with other regions, population pressure, land ownership patterns, and income distribution.

Initially people begin to eat what the land in their immediate surroundings is naturally producing. At this stage, all people of the region eat about the same type of food, because all have the same access to available food supply. Through a very long and slow process of selection and domestication of crop plants and animals, the natural production pattern is altered. In this process, the most favoured crop plants and animals are encouraged and given preference over others. As a consequence, their production begins to dominate the food supply. The consumption pattern begins to mature and is dominated by the most favoured food items. At this stage, people in different income groups begin to eat different quantities and qualities of food because some foods are more expensive than others. Some foods become more expensive because they require more effort to produce or have very low yields.

Bangladesh has a long history of plant and animal domestication. Rice and several lentils and vegetables, which now constitute the primary diet of the people, were domesticated in the region. Bangladesh has plenty of flat and wet areas, which are annually flooded. Agricultural historians believe that it was in such areas of South Asia, that two wild varieties of rice were found growing, from which rice (*oryza sativa*) was derived. Besides having rice, Bangladesh was also a region of primary domestication for peas, gram, beans, taro, yams, bananas, and mangoes. Hence, rice with some lentils and vegetables must have become the primary diet of the people at an early stage and has continued to be so to the present.

Kautilya's *Arthasastra* describes various aspects of the economy during the Chandragupta's empire in the 4th century BC, which extended up to north Bangladesh. In a description of ration distributed to individuals by the state officials, only rice is mentioned (Kangle 1965).There is no reference to wheat and barley, but meat and fish were commonly consumed. The present common diet of the region, consisting of rice, lentils, vegetables, and some meat and fish has persisted, with little alteration, for more than 2,000 years. Rice has become as strongly embedded in the culture of the people as it is in the economy of the nation.

In Bangladesh, land is very fertile. Therefore from very early times it began to attract more people than other parts of South Asia, and it soon became a densely populated region. At present it is 3 times more densely populated than India. A rice diet is ideal for supporting more people because rice yields more per unit area than any other cereal. It is no wonder that rice is so important in the diet of the people. It is only recently, because of increasing population pressure and inadequate supply of rice, that people began to grow and eat wheat in small quantities to compensate for rice shortage. The majority of people in Bangladesh are very poor. They find rice as a staple diet very convenient to cook because it is simply boiled and is ready for consumption. If there is not enough rice to go around for all members of the household, it can be made into a gruel by mixing more water. Hence, it can be stretched more than any other cereal and a given quantity can feed more people.

Culture and the social organization of people have a profound influence on the quantity and quality of food they consume. In Bangladesh, social organization, as in many other developing countries, provides some safety nets against complete starvation. There are a variety of traditional arrangements wherby people are partially fed in times of scarcity. These traditional arrangements were codified by the Mughals in order to make them customary laws (Dasgupta 1987). These arrangements, developed by those who constantly lived in the shadow of hunger, have been described by some as the 'moral economy' of traditional societies. For example, all members of the village have the right to free collection of a number of food and some non-food items that can be exchanged for food from public and private land, when not under cultivation. Hence, landless labourers collect leafy vegetables, berries and fish to supplement their diet. They also collect fodder and various forest products which they can sell or exchange directly for food.

There are also other community traditions such as extended kinship networks that provide support for the relatives during times of food scarcity and save them from complete starvation. For example, married brothers and sisters often live in close proximity and share a common court-yard. In times of scarcity, households of the extended family may borrow food from each other. Short term borrowing of rice is a common practice, but unlike several other items borrowed-rice must always be returned (Rizvi 1987). There is also the custom of sharing the produce of vegetables grown around the house. A large gourd, a bunch of bananas, jackfruit, and mangoes are commonly shared by the households of a joint family. Fish caught and birds and animals hunted by a member of a household are almost always shared with the others. Also, special foods cooked on festive occasions or sometimes just for a change are shared with relatives. For example, sweets and special rice dishes (rice cooked in meat stock and spices or rice cooked in milk and sugar) are shared with close relatives. Among the poor, this constitutes a significant source of nutrition. But with growth of population and settlement this source is rapidly shrinking.

If the bread winner gets sick and unable to work and if there is no stock of food in the house, it is the responsibility of the female head of the household to provide a meal for the immediate family. She often does that by collecting some food from public or private land and by borrowing rice from relatives (Rizvi 1987).

During the time of food scarcity, women of the household often miss lunch to save a little more for the husband and children. In times of acute food shortages, the wife and small children are sometime sent to the wife's parents. Often they are better looked after, if the parents are better off than the husband, and regain lost weight, and return healthier than before.

The religion of people always has a profound influence on their dietary habits. Islam, which is the religion of the vast majority, forbids the eating of pork, but permits the meat of all other animals, if killed in the proper way. Hence, goats, sheep, cattle, fish, and poultry are all consumed freely by those who can afford them. In a densely populated country like Bangladesh, foodgrains provide a cheaper source of calories and protein. If grains are fed to animals they lose a large proportion of their caloric value before they are converted into meat and milk. The general estimate is that 5 calories of vegetable food produce one calorie of meat food (Rao 1982). Animals raised by grazing are not possible because there is little range land in Bangladesh. Hence, a largely vegetarian diet is more sensible despite no religious restrictions. Although development of pig-raising would have been a better alternative for supplying animal protein and fat than cattle, its development is prohibited by religion.

The social and cultural history of people again affects the manner in which food is cooked and its nutritive value. In Bangladesh, as in the rest of the subcontinent, food is cooked to enhance its taste, and not much attention is given to the retention of nutritional values. Mostly food is over cooked, spicy, and fried in oil. In poor households, though, vegetable, fish, and meat dishes, in order to stretch the volume, are always cooked with plenty of water to make thin gravy. Also, to save oil, which is expensive, food is not fried much. Therefore, meat, fish, and vegetable dishes in the poor households retain more nutrients. But even among the poor, chilli-hot and spicy food is preferred. This may be because a small quantity of curry, if it is hot and spicy, is enough for a lot of rice. Spices are also believed to have some medicinal properties. Many people in the hot and humid climate suffer from chronic digestive disorders. Several spices such as garlic, ginger, cumin seeds, and asafoetida seem to help digestion (Chakravarti 1974).

Population pressure is yet another variable that influences food intake, particularly in non-industrial societies. Heavy population pressure leads to smaller and smaller holdings, landlessness, surplus labour, high unemployment, high demand for food, and low wages. All these conditions contribute to food scarcity and make food availability difficult for the poor. The variables that reduce the purchasing power of the landless and small landholders increase the price of food. In Bangladesh, heavy population pressure and consequent scarcity of food have had, until very recently, a significant impact on the food habits of the people. One important change has been increasing consumption of wheat, which was almost absent in the diets of the rich and poor two decades ago. Now it is consumed frequently in both urban and rural areas for at least breakfast because it is cheaper than rice. In some urban households, its consumption even in main meals has commenced. Food habits in general are difficult to change. They are even more difficult to change for rice eaters because rice is very simple to cook. It is simply boiled and eaten directly at all meals with some supplementary dishes to enhance the taste. The preparation of supplementary dishes is always more complex than cooking rice. The preparation of other cereals is more difficult for rice eaters because it requires more elaborate preparation. For example, wheat, maize, or barley have to be first ground into flour, which is made into dough and then only used for making bread or *chappaties* (Chakravarti 1974). For making *chappaties* or *roti*, small quantities of dough are rolled over into round disk-like shapes. Rice eaters have neither the necessary gear nor the expertise for making *chappaties*. Moreover there is also the psychological barrier. Rice eaters think that *chappaties* made from wheat or barley flour are very light and therefore quickly digested, and so one begins to feel hungry again very soon. Before the adoption of wheat, *chappaties* were eaten only when one was sick and unable to digest rice. Hence, switching over to wheat even partially is an admirable change in the diet pattern of the people in Bangladesh.

Yet another change in the diet of the people has been the increasing consumption of potatoes and vegetables. When rice is scarce, in poor households, it is common practice to boil potatoes, squash, and various gourds with rice to increase its volume. Hence, population pressure and consequent food scarcity and high prices have made a significant impression on the food habits of the people in Bangladesh.

In the non-industrial societies, land ownership also has a strong influence on the food intake of people. Large landlords are obviously very well fed and are never hungry. They have sufficient stock of food to depend upon during periods of food scarcity between harvests. Even in the event of a crop failure due to a natural disaster, they have adequate reserve stocks to feed themselves and their families.

Even small landowners are better fed than the landless. By working hard on their own tiny holdings they can often produce just enough for subsistence. But the landless are entirely at the mercy of the landlords and the market. When there is no demand for labour, as is often the case a few months before the harvesting of the main crop, they partially starve. Whenever there is a natural disaster and cropping activities are reduced, the landless starve again. Many landless agricultural labourers say that no matter how hard they work they will be hungry as long as they have no land. Yet land distribution in Bangladesh is consistingly becoming more skewed. More than half the cultivated land is owned by only ten percent of the rural households and about half the rural households have practically no land. The average size of the agricultural holdings has been consistently declining and the number of small holdings is increasing. The area under small holdings now account for a much larger percentage of the area under holdings than it did in 1971. Many small farmers at the same time are being relegated to the rank of landless agricultural labourers. The increasing size of the landless population is very likely to have an adverse effect on the nutritional intake of a large number of households. However, the nutritional surveys, conducted in the 1970s and 1980s, do not seem to indicate that this is happening. Perhaps nutritional intake of the landless households has been prevented from dropping by the Public Food Distribution Program.

The national food supply in non-industrial societies directly affects the food intake of people. This is because, in the case of such societies, the food purchasing power for obtaining food from overseas is very limited. Therefore, when the domestic supply is large and the gap between supply and demand is small, food is relatively cheap and within the reach of the majority of households. When the domestic supply falls far below the requirements, many households cannot afford to buy enough because it is too expensive. In Bangladesh, food supply was inadequate to meet the effective demand throughout the 1970s and early 1980s. The available food was expensive and therefore many poor households could not afford to buy enough for their needs. Therefore, even towards the end of 1980s roughly 45 percent of the population was below the poverty line and was inadequately fed (BBS 1992). Wages have not kept up with the food prices, thereby eroding the food entitlement of landless workers. However, the food supply, as we have already seen in Chapter 4, has increased impressively during the 1980s. Rice production increased by 40 percent in the 1980s, and in 1992 the country became self-sufficient for the first time in its history (FAO 1993). This enormous increase in rice production largely came from the expansion of tube well irrigation followed by the spread of HYRVs. In 1980, tube wells irrigated only 14 percent of all irrigated area, but in 1992 they irrigated 55 percent of irrigated area. Area under shallow tube wells increased at the rate of 30 percent annually in the 1980s. The increased supply has definitely improved the average intake of food and to some extent also the intake of the poor. There has also been a considerable increase in inland and marine fisheries, which has also had a positive impact on the average food intake and the intake of the poor as well. Increase in food supply has a strong positive influence on income distribution as it increases the income not only of the landowners but also of the landless labourers by creating more demand for labour (Mahmud 1990). Increased supply creates more employment for agricultural labourers, village artisans, shopkeepers, and transport workers.

Food deficit in the 1970s and 1980s was made up by imports of foodgrains. Bangladesh in those two decades imported between 7 and 12 percent of its requirements. Some of it was used for the Public Food Distribution Program, which significantly affected the food intake of the poor. It has been found that the program affected the food intake of not only the workers but their whole households, as the food paid for a day's work is enough to feed 3 or 4 individuals.

Composition of average diet and its nutritional value

The average diet in Bangladesh is dominated by rice, pulses, vegetables, and fish, which account for 75 percent of the total quantity of food consumed per day (Table 6.1). These four items account for more than 80 percent of the annual food expenditure in the rural areas and 71 percent in urban areas. There is practically no regional variation in the diet pattern. The urban population appears to be slightly better fed in both quantity and quality. Ahmed et al. (1991), estimated that the average per capita consumption of calories in rural areas was 93 percent of their calorie requirements as against 94 percent in urban areas. The nutritional status of people in terms of calories consumed per capita in rural and urban areas is not very different. But in urban areas people eat a more varied diet. They consume less foodgrains and eat more vegetables, fruits, meat, and fish. After taking sex and age into account, Ahmed et al. (1991) estimated the minimum per capita calorie requirements for Bangladesh to be 2021 for rural and 2075 for urban populations. The higher figure for the urban population is because they have fewer children. The nutritional value of the average diet was not very far below the recommended level for calories and also protein - considering the smaller size and body weight of the people, and the warm climate. A comparison of 1973-74 and 1990-91 HES enables one to see how the nutritional value of the average diet in Bangladesh has changed over time. There appears to be no great change in the composition of the average diet, in the sense that it is still heavily dominated by foodgrains, which account for two-thirds of the daily per capita food intake. Nevertheless, there have been significant changes in the daily intake of nutrients, which indicate considerable improvement in the quality of diet. For example, between 1973-74 and 1990-91, the average daily per capita consumption of calories increased by 15 percent despite considerable population growth. In 1990-91, the average daily per capita calorie consumption in Bangladesh was 2153, which was more than the minimum recommended by Ahmad and Sampath (1991). About 83 percent of the calories are obtained from rice, wheat, and pulses. Another 8 percent are obtained from food items classified as other foods, which are nuts, berries, eggs, and poultry. These foods although consumed in small quantities make an important contribution to the energy consumption of people. Nearly 96 percent of the calories in the average diet still come from vegetable foods.

Table 6.1

Per capita daily consumption of selected nutrients in the average diet in Bangladesh, 1973-74

Food Items	Calories	Protein	Fat	Carotene	(Percentages) Calories	Protein	Fat	Carotene
Rice	1221	26.00	1.77	-	68.40	48.39	11.52	-
Wheat	292	10.00	1.44	24.56	16.36	18.61	9.37	2.38
Potatoes	9	0.15	0.01	2.23	0.50	0.28	0.06	0.22
Pulses	70	5.00	0.44	62.51	3.92	9.31	2.86	6.06
Sugar/gur	43	0.01	0.01	-	2.41	0.02	0.06	-
Edible oils	45	-	5.00	-	2.52	-	32.55	-
Fish	36	5.00	0.36	-	2.02	9.31	2.34	-
Vegetables	26	2.58	0.18	721.00	1.46	4.80	1.17	69.93
Fruits	12	0.19	0.03	64.90	0.67	0.35	0.19	6.29
Milk	25	1.18	2.41	4.60	1.40	2.20	15.69	4.46
Meat	6	0.95	0.30	-	0.34	1.77	1.95	-
Others	85	2.67	3.41	110.00	4.76	4.97	22.20	10.67
TOTAL	1785	53.73	15.36	1031.00	100	100	100	100

1988-89

Food Items	Calories	Protein	Fat	Carotene	(Percentages) Calories	Protein	Fat	Carotene
Rice	1473	32.00	2.13	-	68.42	50.35	9.24	-
Wheat	220	8.00	1.09	18.53	10.22	12.59	4.73	1.47
Potatoes	17	0.57	0.04	8.59	0.79	0.90	0.17	0.68
Pulses	91	6.00	0.58	81.48	4.23	9.44	2.52	6.46
Sugar/gur	16	-	-	-	0.74	-	-	-
Edible oil	56	-	6.20	-	2.60	-	26.91	-
Fish	41	6.00	0.41	-	1.90	9.44	1.78	-
Vegetables	31	3.00	0.21	816.00	1.44	4.72	0.91	64.71
Fruits	15	0.21	0.03	74.60	0.70	0.33	0.13	5.91
Milk	13	0.98	2.00	3.80	0.60	1.54	8.68	3.01
Meat	9	1.40	0.45	-	0.42	2.22	1.95	-
Others	171	5.40	6.90	223.00	7.94	8.50	29.95	17.68
TOTAL	2153	63.56	23.04	1261.00	100	100	100	100

(-) = Negligible. Note: Figures for protein and fat are in grams and those for carotene are in micro-grams

Source: Calculated by the author

The level of protein in the average diet increased by 18 percent during the same period. About 85 percent of protein is still obtained from vegetable food. Fish is the most important source of animal protein. Meat and milk account for about 4 percent of the daily protein intake and vegetables account for a similar amount. Rice continues to supply more than half the daily protein intake, despite its low protein content. This is because a relatively large quantity of rice is consumed in the daily diet.

A certain amount of fat in the daily diet is also necessary for supplying essential fatty acids required by the body. The essential fatty acids are those that the body cannot make. Inadequate supply of essential fatty acids such as linoleic acid causes fatty acid deficiency diseases, a specially in children. It is important that these fatty acids are present in the food because they perform several important functions in the body. The most important perhaps is that they help transport fat soluble vitamins in the body. Despite the importance of fats in the diet, no minimum quantity is generally given in daily dietary allowances. This may be because the body is able to convert excess carbohydrates into fat. However, Gopalan et al. (1984) have prescribed a minimum limit of 15 grams of vegetable oils in the daily diet of individuals to obtain the necessary amounts of essential fatty acids. The average per capita consumption of fat in Bangladesh in 1990-91 was more than 15 grams, hence satisfactory. Most of the fat intake in the daily per capita average diet in Bangladesh comes from vegetable foods. But irrespective of the type, all fats yield the same amount of energy. About 60 percent of the fat in the daily diet comes from edible oils and food items classified as other food. The edible oils that are used freely for frying and seasoning of food, are mustard, til, and peanut oils. Another 16 percent of the fat in the daily diet comes from foodgrains. Only 13 percent of the daily fat intake comes from animal products, namely fish, milk, and meat.

The above discussion indicates that the average per capita daily consumption levels of calories, protein, and fat in Bangladesh are satisfactory. But the average diet appears to be deficient in vitamins, particularly vitamin A. The deficiency of vitamin A can have several crippling effects, the worst of them all being blindness. The problem of blindness is quite common in Bangladesh.

Vitamin A is present in animal foods such as butter, milk, eggs, liver etc. In Bangladesh, because these foods are expensive they are consumed infrequently in small quantities. Vitamin A is not present in vegetable foods, but a substance known as carotene is found in vegetables. Carotene is converted into vitamin A by the body. Therefore, if leafy green vegetables are consumed in sufficient quantities, vitamin A requirements can be easily met. In Bangladesh, people consume a lot of leafy green vegetables besides other vegetables because they go well with rice and are also cheap. Even the poor can afford to consume them in considerable quantities. Some of them are very rich in carotene such as amaranth (*Chaulai sag*), spinach and mustard, radish, yam, and coriander leaves. In rural Bangladesh, some of these can be collected free from the fields or public land. Green chillies, which are also rich in carotene, are also commonly consumed by all. Without leafy greens, vitamin A deficiency would have been much worse.

Despite a notable lack of meat, eggs, and milk in the average diet, nutritionally it is quite satisfactory. Meat, milk, eggs, and fish are consumed only in very small quantities because they are expensive. Nevertheless pulses and vegetables provide adequate protein and vitamins. The protein in pulses is rich in lysine but poor in methionine, while rice protein is poor in lysine but has satisfactory levels of methionine. Hence, a combination of rice and pulses provides enough protein having adequate levels of all essential amino acids.

Except for some vitamins, the average diet in Bangladesh fulfils nutritional requirements fairly well, but the same cannot be said for the common diet of the poor. The quantity of food consumed by the poor — in the five lowest income groups — is considerably smaller than the quantity consumed by the rich - in the five highest income groups. For example, the daily per capita consumption of rice by the poor is less than half the quantity consumed by the rich. Similarly, the daily per capita consumption of vegetables, meat, milk, and edible oils by the poor is much smaller than that by the rich. Since the average diet includes the consumption levels of the rich and the poor, it is quite clear that the consumption levels of the poor are well below the average diet. Hence, the consumption levels of calories, protein, fat, and vitamin A must be well below the recommended levels, because in the average diet they barely meet the recommended levels. This means that in the diet of at least one-third of the population the recommended levels of nutrients are not met. They are, therefore, undernourished.

However the nutritional status of the poor in the rural areas is probably a little better than that portrayed in the HES. The surveys are not able to record several free food items, discussed earlier, which the rural poor are able to collect from their local environment. These free food items are significant sources of protein and vitamins for the poor households.

The poor households consume left over rice from the previous day with pulses or chilli paste. The mid-day meal is cooked and consists of rice with vegetables or fish curry, chillies, and onions. The vegetables are often some variety of gourds grown around the hut or some leafy vegetables either bought or collected free. The evening meal is eaten quite late - about 8 or 9 p.m.- and is very similar to the mid-day meal. Sometimes vegetable curry may be replaced by lentil soup or fish curry.

The well-to-do households in both urban and rural areas have three cooked meals and have more variety and meat and fish dishes. In the urban areas, they consume more wheat than rural households. Often they have *chappaties, paratha, halwa,* or western styled bread made from wheat flour for breakfast.

Although there are large discrepancies between BBS and FAO data concerning changes in the consumption of calories, protein, and fat in the average diet, both sources suggest significant improvements. In 1990-91, the average food intake, as revealed by FAO data, appeared to have improved in quantity but not so much in quality. The average calorie consumption per capita per day for the combined urban and rural population increased by about 4 percent between 1969-71 and 1989-91, but protein consumption increased by only 0.9 percent during the period, based on FAO data. This may be because the level of protein in the average diet at 64 grams was already well above the minimum recommended level. Protein obtained from vegetables sources increased by 6.4 percent but that from animal sources declined. The average calorie consumption in 1989-90 was 98.3 percent of the level recommended by Ahmed et al. (1991) for Bangladesh. While calories and protein intake increased only nominally, the increase in fat intake recorded a phenomenal increase of 34 percent during the same period, most of it coming from vegetable sources. In fact, according to FAO data, per capita fat supply from animal sources declined. The BBS data on the other hand shows a 43 percent increase in per capita meat supply, which is also reflected in per capita consumption of meat in HES data. It is, therefore, quite puzzling to note that per capita fat supply from animal sources declined but per capita supply of meat increased. It only shows that BBS and FAO data are not compatible. The BBS data also indicate that the per capita supply of refined sugar almost doubled during the period, but HES indicate a decline in consumption. This apparent anomaly can perhaps be explained. We noted in the previous chapter that per capita availability of only refined sugar increased but that of gur declined. It is quite possible that sugar intake of urbanites and rural rich increased several fold, but for the majority of the poor the consumption of sugar declined because it became more expensive. Hence, average actual consumption declined despite an increase in average supply.

Despite some discrepancies in the BBS data, there are some important agreements in the BBS data on per capita availability of several food items and HES data on actual consumption. HES data show that average consumption of fruits, vegetables, meat, and fish has increased, which is strongly supported by BBS per capita availability data. The important point to note is that all sources of data — BBS, FAO, and HES — indicate some increase in the average calorie consumption. Many nutritionists now believe that if the calorie requirements of individuals are satisfied there is a good chance that protein and mineral requirements will also be met. Therefore, it is very encouraging indeed to note that the average calorie consumption in Bangladesh has been increasing and is now almost about the recommended level.

Changes in food consumption patterns

Average diet and actual food consumption patterns in Bangladesh have undergone significant changes for the better not only for the rich but also for the poor. Since independence, six HES in 1973-74, 1981-82, 1983-84, 1985-86, 1988-89, and 1991-92 have been conducted, which provide a wealth of reliable data for analyzing the nature of food consumption pattern in Bangladesh. While National Food Balance Sheets (NFBS) provide a general picture of per capita availability of calories, protein, and fat obtained from major food items and expected per capita consumption, the HES provide more accurate information on actual consumption of food. The HES also give information about monthly expenditure on different food items and the quantity consumed. Hence, they permit analysis of quantity and quality of food consumed by individuals and households in different income groups. The increases in per capita expenditure on food at constant prices indicate increases in the quantity consumed or improvements in the quality of diet of individuals and households in different income groups.

The NFBS and HES data both display an improvement in the quantity and quality of average food intake in both rural and urban areas of Bangladesh. Between the averages of two four year periods, i.e., 1969-73 and 1986-90, per capita supply of calories and fat increased significantly but that of protein remained more or less the same (Table 6.1). The per capita supply of cereals, meat, and sugar increased by 12, 42, and 100 percent respectively. It is rather puzzling to note that while per capita supply of meat increased by 42 percent, it made no impact on per capita supply of protein. The per capita supply of meat in absolute terms increased only from 2.3 to 3.3 kg per year or just 9 grams per day, which is just a tiny piece of meat providing only 2.25 grams of protein. Similarly, the per capita supply of eggs increased by 100 percent, but in absolute terms it increased from 9 eggs to only 14 eggs per year per person. That is, on an average, just about one egg per month. It appears that meat and eggs have not yet become important sources of protein for the majority of the population. The per capita supply of milk, another important source of protein, remained unchanged over the period. It means that the bulk of the protein supply still comes from vegetable sources. Cereals and pulses are still the main sources of protein for the majority of the people in Bangladesh, because meat, fish, eggs, and milk are too expensive for them to afford. Because per capita supply of cereals and pulses increased only marginally, the protein intake on the average remained unchanged.

There seems to be some accord in per capita supply of food for domestic consumption and actual consumption in Bangladesh. The HES in 1988-89 indicate that per capita monthly expenditure on food compared with 1973-74 increased by 22 percent in real terms. At the same time, the share of foodgrains in per capita monthly expenditure on food declined during the period but the quantity consumed has increased by 12 percent. This means that household incomes have increased significantly in real terms. Therefore, despite consuming larger quantities of foodgrains, the proportion of the food budget spent on them is smaller. It appears that a higher percentage of the food budget is now spent on vegetables, fruits, and edible oils. The per capita supply of fat during the period in Bangladesh increased by 34 percent, mostly from vegetable sources (FAO 1992). In fact, increased per capita supply of calories, protein, and fat all came from vegetable sources - increased supply of foodgrains, fruits, and vegetables (FAO 1992). The FAO and HES data both show that food intake by individuals has increased in quantity and improved in quality. It is important to note that this change occurred in both urban and rural areas and also for individuals in low income groups. The 1988-89 HES shows that the percentage of the population in the lowest expenditure group has declined very significantly compared with 1973-74, indicating that the nutritional status of the population in Bangladesh has increased not only for the rich but also for the poor.

The proportion of food expenditure increased on potatoes, fish, vegetables, fruits and milk, but it declined on foodgrains, pulses, sugar, edible oils, and meat. One can understand the decline in the share of food expenditure on foodgrains, which indicates some prosperity and improvement in the diet, but the declining share of food expenditure on sugar, edible oils, and meat is hard to explain. If we assume that the reduced share of food expenditure on foodgrains reflects increased incomes, then this increase must also be reflected in the increased expenditure on sugar, oils, and meat, because increased prosperity generally leads to increased consumption of these three items. But this did not happen in Bangladesh. Instead, improvement of diet has been attained by increasing the consumption of potatoes, fish, vegetables, and fruits, which appears to be a better and less expensive alternative.

The relative share of major food items in monthly per capita food expenditure changed little, with the exception of edible oils and items reported together as other food. The percentage point change was less than 3 for all items, and for most it was within plus or minus 2 percentage points. The quantity consumed for all food items increased, except for wheat, sugar, and milk. However, with the exception of potatoes and other food items, the percentage increase was less than 50 for all food items. In order to show both the changes in the quantity consumed and the share in the food expenditure, all food items were classified into four categories. There were only 5 items in the first category, namely potatoes, fruits, vegetables, other food items, and fish, which increased in the relative share of monthly per capita food expenditure and also quantity consumed (Figure 6.1). In the second category, there were 5 food items, which recorded an increase in the quantity consumed but a decline in the relative share of per capita monthly food expenditure. The third category represents wheat and sugar, which declined both in relative share and quantity consumed. In the last category there is only milk, which declined in the quantity consumed but slightly increased in its relative share.

The changes in per capita consumption of various food items, displayed in (Figure 6.1), clearly show an improvement in per capita consumption of food. Despite the fact that vegetables, fruits, potatoes, and fish are relatively more expensive than foodgrains, people are spending a higher percentage of their food budget on them, because they are more nutritious and make food more tasty. This can only happen when there is a significant increase in per capita income. People use additional income to first fulfil their basic foodgrain needs adequately, then use any extra for improving the taste and nutritional value of the diet. This appears to have happened in Bangladesh. The quantity of foodgrains consumed has increased, but the share of monthly food expenditure on foodgrains has declined, indicating clearly a rise in per capita income and food expenditure. Rice, pulses, meat, oils, and other food items have all recorded an increase in per capita consumption but a drop in the share of monthly food expenditure. The changes in consumption patterns, as displayed in the second category, again confirm a rise in per capita expenditure on food in real terms. Although people increased expenditure on the food items given in the second category, the increase was much less than the overall increase in monthly food expenditure. This implies that increased food expenditure was spent more on so-called luxury food items to enhance the taste and nutritional value of food, such as those given in the first category.

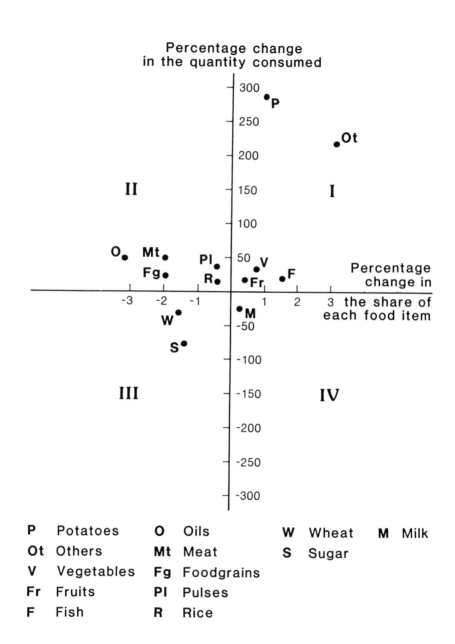

Percentage change in the quantity consumed

II

I

III

IV

Percentage change in the share of each food item

P	Potatoes	O	Oils	W	Wheat	M	Milk
Ot	Others	Mt	Meat	S	Sugar		
V	Vegetables	Fg	Foodgrains				
Fr	Fruits	Pl	Pulses				
F	Fish	R	Rice				

Figure 6.1   Changes in average diet between 1974 and 1989

The consumption of wheat and sugar declined both in quantity and relative share. We have already seen that wheat is not a favoured foodgrain in Bangladesh. The shortage of rice led to the introduction of wheat, which people began to eat reluctantly. In the 1980s, rice output increased by about 32 percent and the rice shortage was wiped off. Therefore people switched back to rice and reduced wheat consumption. This is displayed in Figure 6.1. Per capita rice consumption increased and that of wheat declined.

Sugar supply in Bangladesh increased in recent years but at the expense of gur. The per capita availability of white sugar increased considerably but that of gur declined. Hence, sugar became a more expensive item for a large majority of households. Perhaps its consumption increased for the rich but the average declined.

Milk is not an important item in the average diet of Bangladeshis. It is consumed only in small quantities with tea or it is used for making some sweets, which are consumed by the majority infrequently only on special occasions. Perhaps the price of milk increased more than the per capita expenditure on food. Therefore, people, in order to buy even a reduced quantity of milk, had to increase expenditure on milk more than the total increase on monthly food budget .

The overall changes in per capita food consumption are very encouraging. The foodgrain needs on the average appear to have been adequately met due to increased per capita income and supply. The effort is now towards improving the taste and nutritional quality of the diet. This claim is supported not only by the HES but also by per capita availability and production data. This is indeed a remarkable achievement for a country so densely populated and so frequently afflicted by natural disasters.

Seasonal variations in food intake

The temperatures are mild enough throughout the year in Bangladesh to permit year-round cultivation of crops, but the sowing and harvesting of crops depend very much on the timing of monsoon rains. Minor rains come in the months of February and March, when the planting of the *Aus* rice crop begins. The main rice crop (*Aman*) is planted at the beginning of the summer monsoon rains, in the months of July and August. Food supply, particularly in the rural areas, depends on the harvesting seasons of the main food crops. Before the harvesting of each major foodgrain crop (*Aman, Aus, Boro* and wheat), which is the lean periods, there is a significant drop in the supply. During the lean period food prices rise, and therefore landless labourers and small holders, who purchase either all or part of their food requirements from the market, have to reduce food intake because food is expensive. Ironically, the incomes of the landless labourers also drop during the lean periods, because there is no work in the fields for a few weeks before harvesting begins. The available labour supply becomes higher then the prevailing demand, therefore, wages drop not only for the little agricultural work that might be available but also for non-agricultural work. Mahmud (1990) has clearly shown that increase in staple food supply in the market has a strong influence on the determination of real income distribution due to increased employment, higher wages, and lower prices. In the lean seasons when the supply of food, work opportunities, and wages are all down and food prices are up, the food purchasing power of the poor, particularly, is badly eroded. The poor suffer a real loss of entitlement to food. Therefore, the bulk of the adjustment to reduced food supply is made by the poor. The rich can afford to pay higher prices for food and continue to consume the usual quantity and quality of food. When food begins to take a higher proportion of their income, they can reduce expenditure on less essential items such as entertainments and clothing, and save less. The food entitlement failure arises due to the effects of higher food prices on reduced real wages.

There are two lean periods in a year, when food stocks are at their lowest, food prices at their highest, and employment opportunities and wages at their lowest. The first lean period is in June and July before the harvesting of *Aus* and planting of *Aman.* The *Aman* crop, especially transplanted *Aman*, cannot be planted until late July or August due to insufficient depth of water in the fields. The second lean period is in October and November, before the harvesting of *Aman*. Again, a similar situation prevails in this period as in June and July. Therefore, due to entitlement failure, the food intake of individuals drops substantially during these two lean periods. Bayliss-Smith (1981) worked out monthly average intake of food per head for a number of households and found a strong seasonal trend. Intake of vitamins and micro nutrients also vary seasonally, because many fruits are consumed only in the seasons when they are available. For example, mangoes, jackfruits, lychies, and pineapples are available only in the summer months, while guavas and oranges are only available in winter. Intake of vitamin A and C is high in the summer months because a larger variety of fruits are available and are relatively cheap. It is also noted that particular foodgrains are consumed in different seasons because of seasonality in cereal supply. Rice is consumed mainly during the months following the harvest of *Aman, Aus,* and *Boro* - from July to February. From March to June rice is supplemented with wheat and potatoes. However, in some districts with the expansion of irrigation three rice crops in a year are produced, which has practically eliminated seasonality in cereal supply in recent years.

Nutritional status of mothers and children also changes seasonally. It drops to its lowest in August to October, when the main rice crop is in the fields. The *Aus* stock may still be available but there is no work in these two months and rice prices are high. Food purchasing power drops to its lowest.

Besides seasonality of supply, seasonality of infectious diseases also affects nutritional status of the poor, particularly children. Diarrhoea, for example, is more prevalent in the months of March and September. It causes anorexia, reduces food holding capacity, and adversely affects digestion. Food intake is further reduced because when adults are sick they cannot earn income. Here again, the poor suffer more because more frequently they eat left over stale food. They also shop around for cheap vegetables and meat that are often partially spoiled.

The above discussion clearly reveals that the burden of seasonal fluctuations in food supply and sickness is heavily borne by the poor landless labourers and small farmers.

Gender bias in food intake

In Islamic culture particularly, women play a subordinate role in society in almost all respects. They are expected not to expose their face and other parts of the body, not to express their views in a conversation among men, not to go to entertainments and participate in games and sports as frequently as men. They are, therefore, more housebound. They get less education and are deprived of many social and cultural activities that are essential for the development of personality. This relative suppression of women also exists in other traditional Asian, African, and Middle Eastern societies, but in all these regions it is more prominent among the Muslims. In the poor households, partly because of their subordinate role in society, they are discriminated against in the allocation of available food. Women eat only after feeding the working or adult males in the household. Therefore, when food is scarce, women often get less to eat.

Gender bias in intra-family distribution of food in South Asia, Africa, and the Middle East has been reported by several researchers. Some studies on the theme also exist for Bangladesh. However, the results are conflicting. Chen et al. (1981) reported the existence of a much higher percentage of malnourished girls than boys in the age group of 1 to 5. Abdullah and Wheeler (1985) noted no difference in the proportion of malnourishment among boys and girls under the age of 5. They also found that food intake of women remained unchanged throughout the year but it was below that of men. They also felt that food intake of women on average was quite right for their needs, because women are smaller in size and weight and generally do not participate in hard field labour. Their hard manual work is only rice husking and bringing water from streams or wells. Sen (1984) noted that girls under the age of 6 bore the brunt of food shortages that followed the 1978 floods. It has been noted that in times of acute food scarcity, even in the female-headed households, gender bias in food allocation against girls exists in Bangladesh (Sen 1984, Bairage 1986, Pryer 1987). Harris (1990) found that food intake of women in central Bangladesh was only 15 percent less than that of men, which is commensurate with the level recommended by FAO and WHO. About 2/3 of the intra-household energy intake of adult women and children aged 4-6 in statistically accounted for by the absolute intake of adult males. So, only 1/3 of the variation may be due to other factors. Despite the contradictory nature of the results, some explanations for gender bias in food allocation is provided. The economic explanation, which is the most common, states that adult males are fed more because they work hard and bring money to buy food or bring food directly in the form of wages for the entire household. If they are not fed adequately, they will not have the physical strength required to get employment in a highly competitive labour market. Women and children stay home and do lighter jobs, if any. Therefore, to feed men a little more than women and children is an efficient survival strategy. Greenough (1982) provides a strong social reason for gender bias in the allocation of food. The continuity of the family depends on the male adults, and continuity provides several social and economic advantages. Older households command more power and respect in the village. For example, the village headman is generally from the oldest household. The village headman and his entire household enjoy several economic advantages in a village community.

Thus gender bias in the intra-household allocation of available food, if it exists, although cruel, can be defended on both social and economic grounds.

Food consumption in different income groups

Earlier in this chapter we made a passing comment, without presenting any data, that the quantity and quality of food consumed by individuals have improved during the reference period among both the rich and the poor. In this section, we examine the pattern of food consumption in the low and high income groups in order to see whether the food intake of the poor has really improved over time.

The proportion of total expenditure on food has declined for both the rich and the poor. For the three lowest income groups, the percentage of total expenditure on food dropped from 75.4 in 1973-74 to 73 percent in 1988-89. It is not a spectacular drop, have nevertheless significant. It means that even the poor are spending a relatively smaller share of the total expenditure on food. This could have happened due to either a drop in food prices or a real rise in incomes. Also, it could have been the result of a drop in real incomes and expenditure, compelling people to curtail expenses on some expensive food items in order to save for other necessities. In that case the drop would have been relative and also absolute. But, in fact, per capita income in Bangladesh has increased in real terms during the period. Therefore, a drop in the share of total expenditure on food reflects only a relative decline in expenditure on food and not an absolute decline. We have already noted that per capita expenditure on food increased by 22 percent in real terms during the period. This could not have happened without a real increase in per capita income. Hence, a smaller share of total expenditure on food suggests an improvement in the well-being of the people.

The share of total expenditure on food declined much more for the rich than for the poor. For the three highest income groups, the percentage of total expenditure on food dropped from about 66 percent in 1973-74 to 47 in 1990-91. It suggests that a much bigger proportion of economic growth went to the rich. Their incomes increased much faster than food prices and also faster than the incomes of the poor, indicating a widening gap between the rich and the poor.

The quantity of food consumed by individuals in the five highest expenditure groups is two and a half times more than per capita consumption in the five lowest expenditure groups. Even the per capita consumption of rice in the five highest expenditure groups is two and a half times higher than the quantity of rice for the five lowest expenditure groups. A much wider gap between the rich and the poor exists in per capita consumption of more expensive food items such as meat, milk, and fruits. The per capita consumption in the three highest expenditure groups for milk, sugar, meat, and fruits is 19, 12.5, 10, and 8 times more respectively than in the three lowest expenditure groups. The difference in per capita consumption of

146

vegetables and fish is not that large, because the poor get some portion of their supply from free collection.

The above discussion clearly shows that the rich not only consume a larger quantity of food but also more nutritious food than the poor. Among several variables that may affect future food consumption levels in Bangladesh, changes in food supply, per capita income, income distribution, and population growth appear to be the major determinants. We have already noted that expenditure on food in real terms increased during the reference period and that it was due to increase in incomes across the board. Per capita food supply has also increased for all major food items and this trend is very likely to continue for some time. There is also considerable unutilized potential in fisheries. More attention to the development of fisheries will certainly make a significant contribution to food supply.

Along with these changes, there is impressive progress in population control. Between 1975 and 1991, the use of contraceptives by eligible women increased from 5 percent to more than 40 percent, which is impressive indeed for a Muslim society. Therefore, population growth is bound to drop quite significantly in the near future, helping to raise per capita food supply faster than in the 1970s and 1980s. Furthermore, the industrial sector is expanding quite rapidly. Public and private investment in manufacturing doubled between 1975 and 1991. The value added in the manufacturing sector increased by 300 percent during the 1980s, and employment in manufacturing also increased significantly. The growth in manufacturing will help increase food purchasing power of the people by providing more employment. The development of export-oriented industries will increase the food purchasing power of the country from overseas.

Summary

The common diet in Bangladesh consists of rice, lentils, vegetables, and some fish. This diet has persisted — with little alteration — for centuries. Rice can support more people per unit of land than any other cereal and therefore it has continued to be the most popular staple. However, increasing population pressure and food scarcity have compelled people to change their food habits and consume more wheat and potatoes than before.

During the two decades under review the average food intake in Bangladesh improved in both quantity and quality. Although there are big differences in the BBS and FAO estimates of changes in the consumption of calories, protein, and fat in the average diet, both show a positive change. About 2/3 of the protein still comes from cereals and only 1/3 from fish, pulses, and vegetables. The consumption of foodgrains has been increasing in the lower income groups but beginning to decline in the high income groups. The consumption of fish and vegetables has been increasing in all income groups. The nutritional quality of the average diet and the average diet in each income group seems to be quite satisfactory compared to the recommended level and have been improving over time.

The quantity and quality of food intake drop significantly during the two lean periods, that is, before harvesting of *Aus* crop and before the harvesting of *Aman* crop. Within a given household females are often discriminated against in the distribution of available food among the members. Whenever there is a scarcity of food, women sacrifice and settle for the smallest share of the available food. However, the social organization provides some safety nets during scarcity whereby people are partially fed. Such traditions reduce mortality due to starvation.

7 Hunger and undernutrition

Definitions and alternative methods of hunger estimation

Hunger and undernutrition may be defined as a condition in which an individual does not have the resources to acquire the minimum recommended daily calorie requirement (MRDCR). In the countries where no nutrition or household expenditure surveys are conducted, it is impossible to estimate precisely the extent of hunger and undernutrition. Nevertheless, some idea of the prevalence of hunger in a country or a region can be gained from demographic data. For example, high infant mortality and morbidity are good indicators of undernutrition. National food balance sheets are also frequently used to get some idea of aggregate hunger. In food balance sheets, one estimates the actual amount of food available for human consumption in a given year. This takes into account the stock of food brought forward from the previous year, production during the year, imports and exports, food fed to livestock, food wasted during storage and transportation, seed kept for the next crop, and the stock of food carried over into next year, to get the actual quantity available for human consumption. Once such estimates are made for each food item in a given country, the food consumed by the human population can be converted into calories, protein, and other nutrients. The supply of these can then be compared with requirements. But food balance sheets give only a rough estimate of average intake of food, because it is assumed that available food is uniformly distributed among the entire population.

Anthropometry, the science of measuring the human body and its various parts, provides yet another alternative for measuring undernutrition or the nutritional status of a given population. Although human physical growth and development may be affected by genetics, health and sanitation standards, and the presence or absence of vitamins in the diet, they are most certainly affected by the intake of calories and protein. Therefore, weight, height, muscle, and fat of the human body for age and sex, when compared to some standard figure, give clues about adequate or inadequate calorie and protein intake. It is supposed to be a low cost and highly accurate method (Foster 1992). It does not require a highly trained staff. Despite these advantages, it has not become popular in the Third World countries, where the need for the assessment of hunger and undernutrition is most urgent.

A reasonably accurate picture of undernutrition and overnutrition can be gained only from the data collected in Household Expenditure Surveys and Household Nutrition Surveys. The Household Expenditure Surveys in Bangladesh collect data on about 1500 expenditure and income items. The 1989-90 HES covered 5,675 households (urban 1,871 and rural 3,804), which gave a coverage of 31,571 people, and the same coverage was maintained in 1991-92. The HES of 1991-92 was spread over the entire 12 month period. The data were collected by interviewers and diary keepers, who were given intensive training at BBS, Dhaka, and 22 Regional Statistical Offices. They were, therefore, adequately trained for the job. Further, when they were working in the field, their work was frequently checked by Regional Statistical Officers for accuracy. The diary system, introduced recently, is for collecting information on expenditure on basic necessities. Under this system, details of purchase and consumption of food and beverage items are collected daily for an entire month from the sample households. HES data give a break down of expenditure on various food items, total food, and non-food items for households in 16 income classes. Hence, it is possible to work out how much a household spends on food, what quantity of the most common regional food can be bought for that amount, and what nutritional status members in the household enjoy. However, HES data do not permit an estimation of intra-household differences in food intake.

In Bangladesh, Household Nutrition Surveys (HNS) are also conducted, but at irregular intervals, and only a couple have been conducted since independence. The HNS, therefore, are not suitable for analyzing hunger and undernutrition trends. Further, the HNS has a much smaller coverage, but it gives data on the actual quantity of food consumed by households. Therefore, HNS data make possible more accurate direct measurement of hunger and undernutrition than HES data.

In Bangladesh, fortunately, HES data are available for a fairly long time, and their quality has consistently improved over the years. Therefore, HES data permit estimation of the extent of hunger and undernutrition in Bangladesh, and trends in these over time. The first HES survey in independent Bangladesh was conducted in 1973-74, and the latest in 1991-92. But at the time of writing this chapter (April 1995) only few summary tables for 1991-92 HES were available. Therefore, some of the analysis in this chapter is based on the 1988-89 HES report. For changes in food poverty (throughout this study food poverty, hunger, and undernutrition have been used interchangeably) the HES data for the years 1973-74, 1981-82, 1983-84, 1985-86, 1988-89, and 1991-92 were used. Although HES surveys were also conducted in the years 1974-75, 1975-76, 1976-77, 1977-78, and 1978-79, the detailed reports for these five years were never published due to long delays in data processing and some doubts about the quality of data (BBS 1991). It is perhaps because of the poor quality of the data that no mention is made of the proportion of the food poor population in these years in any of the HES reports between 1981-82 and 1991-92. Therefore, for reasons of greater reliability we used only six HES years, as mentioned above, for the present analysis.

The households whose per capita expenditure on food is less than that required to purchase MRDCR from the most common diet of the region are classified as hungry. But MRDCR for growth, maintenance, and normal activities has been vigorously debated in recent years (Sukhatme 1977, 1978, and 1981; Dandekar 1981; Gopalan 1983; Achaya 1983; Srinivasan 1983; among many others). It will, therefore, be inappropriate to proceed further without discussing the main points of the debate.

As a result of a better understanding of the energy requirements of the human body, the MRDCR figures now recommended are significantly lower than those in the 1950s (Sukhatme and Margen 1982; Gopalan et al. 1981; FAO 1977). It is stressed that an average MRDCR figure for adults may be too high for some individuals in the same category, because they may need much less energy. Just as some machines are more energy efficient than other, some humans are also more efficient converters of food into food energy. Sukhatme (1977) argues that the cut-off line for minimum calorie requirement should be (m- 2sd), where m is the mean requirement of a population and sd is the standard deviation representing inter-individual variations. Sukhatme (1978) argues that not only intake but also requirement for a given individual vary from day to day. Therefore, some individuals can tolerate a significant drop in intake without loosing body weight and change in life style, for some time. This is achieved through the homoeostasis (regulatory) mechanism in human the body. If the food intake is inadequate for a considerable time the individual will begin to loose body weight. Following this line of argument, Sukhatme (1978) uses the cutoff point of 2300 calories per consumer unit or 1900 calories per capita per day to define hunger, which is based on an assumed 15 percent coefficient of variation in requirements per consumer unit. The efficiency of food varies within individuals and is self regulated by homoeostasis, which maintains a balance between consumption and replenishment of nutrients (Sukhatme and Margen 1982). This viewpoint has been strongly criticised on the grounds that it was based on inadequate experimental work (Achaya 1983, Gopalan 1983, Kakwani 1989). Further, it relies heavily on the principle of the adaptation of human body to a lower intake and not on physiological need. It is like saying that the scant clothing the poor wear in winter is an indication that they do not suffer from exposure to winter cold. Millions of poor suffer from exposure to cold in winter because they cannot afford adequate clothing, but over time their bodies adapt to what they can afford. Nevertheless, many still die from influenza and pneumonia because of inadequate protection from cold. This, therefore, does not mean that they do not need clothes or that what they can afford is adequate.

There are several other problems in measuring hunger from grouped data, whether it is for income or expenditure or average calorie consumption. The first problem arises because all individuals in an income class arc treated as equal. No distinction is made between those whose income is close to the upper limit and those who are at the bottom end. Those who are at the upper end of the critical

151

expenditure class may be very nearly able to meet their minimum nutritional requirement and may not be really undernourished. Secondly, treatment of all members in a class as being at the same nutritional level completely ignores the individual differences in intake and requirement. Some individuals who may be able to fulfil their minimum requirement by consuming less than the minimum recommended intake, because of their smaller size or weight, will also be classified as hungry. Thirdly, a lot of poor people in traditional societies in rural areas are entitled to collect several edible items free, which may not have much market value, but nevertheless significantly add to the nutritional intake of the poor. Even if we accept that most of the items of free collection are recorded by interviewers, the conversion of such items into money would involve inaccuracies. This problem is partly overcome by using average calorie consumption rather than minimum expenditure. But the average expenditure on food by income classes is the only information available in Bangladesh for the estimation of hunger trends. Therefore, one has no choice but to use HES data for estimating hunger and undernutrition.

The MRDCR allowance takes into account basal metabolic rate (BMR), energy lost immediately after a meal, and the minimum energy required for physical activities. The BMR is the energy required for the internal activities of the body, which are heart beat, blood circulation, kidney functions, and functioning of lungs etc. The major flaw in this thinking is that BMR is the same for all individuals having the same body weight, height, age, and sex. The experimental work carried out in the early 1980s revealed, although inadequately, that BMR varies for individuals having the same visible characteristics. However, the concept of a variable BMR would make the setting of MRDCR for a reasonably large population impossible, because such data is neither available nor will ever be possible to obtain at the national scale. Yet another problem in the usage of MRDCR is its concern with calories alone, but undernutrition is not simply inadequate intake of calories. The lack of other major nutrients also contributes significantly to undernutrition, such as vitamin A, iron and vitamins of the B group. Therefore, Gopalan (1983) suggests a least cost balanced diet for estimating the extent of undernutrition.

How much hunger and undernutrition in Bangladesh?

Bangladesh employs the head-count ratio for estimating hunger and undernutrition in the country. The head-count ratio is simply the percentage of population below a defined level of nutritional intake. The head-count ratio does not make any distinction between mild and severe forms of undernutrition. Within the proportion of the population that is said to be suffering from undernutrition, there are large inter-individual variations, which are exposed by the Sen index. Nevertheless, the head-count ratio is the most commonly used measure of hunger and undernutrition. In Bangladesh, the BBS uses two MRDCR levels to define undernutrition and extreme undernutrition, described later in this section. Further, as far as trends in hunger and undernutrition are concerned, both measures (head-count and the Sen index) give identical results (Ahluwalia 1985). For the purpose of measuring undernutrition or food poverty, Bangladesh employs the MRDCR level given by the WHO/FAO expert group for South Asia. It is 2,122 calories, when weighted for the age and occupational profile of Bangladesh. The World Bank also used the same calorie limits for estimating undernutrition in Bangladesh (World Bank 1986). Ahmad, Khan, and Sampath (1991) used the MRDCR level which is just 100 calories lower than the limit used by the BBS and the World Bank, even after adjusting it for age, sex, and occupation. Such a small difference in calories is not likely to make any significant difference in per capita expenditure, therefore, in the proportion of the population undernourished. Therefore, the MRDCR limits used by the BBS are quite appropriate for estimating undernutrition in the country. Furthermore, the BBS has used the same MRDCR limits for all the nine HESs, which makes comparisons over time possible.

In Bangladesh, those whose nutritional intake does not provide them with 2,122 calories, are classified as undernourished. Extreme undernutrition is defined as 85 percent of 2,122 calories or 1,805 calories. The next step in estimating hunger is to calculate the minimum expenditure necessary to acquire 2,122 calories from the most common diet of the poor. The BBS estimates the required level of per capita expenditure for each of the two MRDCR levels, taking into account the retail prices of food items that constitute the most common minimum diet in the country. In 1988-89, the estimated per capita expenditure for a 2,122 calories daily diet was 370 takas per month for rural and 500 takas for urban areas. Monthly minimum per capita expenditures for extreme undernutrition or hard core food poverty for rural and urban areas were estimated to be 303 and 311 takas respectively. The households where monthly per capita expenditure was less than the defined limits were regarded as suffering from undernutrition or extreme undernutrition.

In 1991-92, HES data revealed that actual food intake of 47 percent of the population was not adequate for providing 2,122 calories (MRDCR). They were, therefore, regarded as undernourished (Table 7.1). The majority of the undernourished population, just like the total population, lives in the rural areas (Table 7.1). But in relative terms, the percentage of the population undernourished is practically the same in both rural and urban areas. There is a greater concentration of extreme hunger in the rural areas, where it is 2.1 percentage points higher than in urban areas, despite the fact that food is more expensive in urban areas, and one needs a slightly higher per capita expenditure for the same MRDCR diet. A lower level of extreme undernutrition in urban areas is partly explained by higher wages, higher employment opportunities, and subsidized distribution of food through ration shops in cities and towns. South Asia has the largest concentration of hunger and undernutrition in the world. It is often believed that within the region the highest concentration of hunger is in Bangladesh, but this is not true. In 1985-86, the percentage of hungry in Bangladesh was the same as the average for South Asia (World Bank 1990). In 1991-92, the percentage dropped by another 2.4 percentage points, and was almost 2 percentage points lower than the average for South Asia.

Table 7.1
Hunger and undernutrition over time

| HES years | Percent of population consuming less than 2,122* calories per person daily | |
	Rural	Urban
1973-74	82.9	81.4
1981-82	73.8	66.0
1983-84	57.0	66.0
1985-86	51.0	56.0
1988-89	47.8	47.6
1991-92	47.6	46.7

* A person whose daily intake of food is below 2,122 calories
is regarded as suffering from hunger and undernutrition
Source: BBS Household Expenditure Surveys

Hunger trends

An extensive literature on hunger and food poverty already exists for Bangladesh (Rahman 1985, Boyace 1985, Rehman and Haque 1988, Dayal 1988, Osmani 1990, Khan 1990 among others). The majority of these studies are concerned with hunger trend in the country, especially since independence. But the results of these studies are inconsistent. For example, some writers maintain that hunger and undernutrition have worsened over time and that increased food production did not make much impact on reduction of hunger (Khan 1990, Osmani 1991). But there are others who support the view that reduction in hunger and undernutrition as revealed by HES is real, although may be treated with some caution, because of changes in the methods of data collection since 1983-84 HES (World Bank 1987, BBS 1988, Rahman and Haque 1988). The inconsistencies in the results are due to three main reasons. First, the production data for the periods before and after independence are not strictly comparable due to significant changes in collection methods. Therefore, those who have used data spreading over both periods have arrived at somewhat unreliable results. Second, we have already seen in Chapter 1 that when Bangladesh was under Pakistan, not much investment was made in agricultural and other developments. Therefore, from the mid 1970s, after the temporary dislocation of agriculture was fully restored, food production really began to increase at an accelerated rate. Third, most studies, published up to the 1990s, used only data up to 1983-84, and therefore they could not include the period of the most vibrant growth of food production and wages in the history of Bangladesh.

The general trend in hunger and undernutrition in Bangladesh is similar to that in the world and South Asia. The absolute numbers and the proportion of the population undernourished have both consistently declined since independence (Table 7.1). The incidence of undernutrition almost halved between 1971 and 1991. The first HES, conducted in 1973-74 in independent Bangladesh, revealed that more than 80 percent of the population in the new country was undernourished. The results directed the government's immediate attention to the most serious problem the country was facing, and helped in arranging development priorities. As a result, the eradication of hunger and undernutrition received a high priority in development planning. Most of the 1970s were spent in the development and expansion of facilities required for increasing food production. Therefore, large increases were recorded in irrigation facilities, area under HYVs, use and production of fertilizers and insecticides, and multiple cropping, which continued into the 1980s. Although these developments began to have some impact on food output from the mid 1970s, most of the increase in food production came in the 1980s. Rice production in 1992 stood at 18.25 million tons, which was 84 percent more than the level in 1972-73. Besides — as we have already seen in chapter 4 — rice production and per capita availability of other food items (including fruits, vegetables, and meat) also increased considerably during the period. Thus, food production and per capita availability figures strongly support the declining trend in hunger and undernutrition as revealed in the HES surveys. Between the first and the last HESs, conducted in 1973-74 and 1991-92, the proportion of undernourished dropped from 83 to only 47. This is a very significant drop in hunger and undernutrition. The biggest drop in the proportion of the population hungry was between 1981-82 and 1983-84, when it dropped by 17 percentage points. Since then the decline has been consistent but much slower.

Although there appears to be a strong inverse relationship between food output and undernutrition, increased food availability does not guarantee increased consumption, unless there is a simultaneous increase in incomes and/or improvement in income distribution. The HES and national account data on income and expenditure show that both have increased significantly (BBS 1991). Since 1973-74, per capita income and expenditure, at constant prices, have both been increasing at the annual rate of 1.5 and 0.5 percent respectively (BBS 1995). In 1973-74, per capita income at constant prices was 4,920 takas and in 1988-98 it was 6,205. Similarly, annual per capita expenditure, at constant prices, rose from 5,199 to 5,615 takas during the same period.

The government's efforts to reduce undernutrition in the country were somewhat marred by a lack of improvement in income distribution. It is unfortunate that the gap between the rich and the poor has increased somewhat in recent years (Table 7.2). The share of the lowest 5 percent of the households in the total income dropped slightly between 1973-74 and 1991-92. Also, income accruing to households in the lowest four deciles dropped from 18.3 to 17.5 percent between 1973-74 and 1991-92. On the other hand, the share of income accruing to households in the top 5 percent income class increased by 2.45 percentage points. Also, the share of households in total income in the highest income decile increased

155

by 0.8 percentage points. While the share in total income of the households in the highest income group increased, the share of those in the lowest income groups declined, indicating widening gap between the rich and the poor . This, of course, does not mean that the poor are now worse off than before. The household incomes of the poor also increased but not as much as the income of the rich. The increase in inequality that occurred between 1973-74 and 1991-92 was too small to alter the main results of the surveys. If the income of the poor and the rich had increased in the same proportion, some more households would have reached MRDCR, and the percentage of the population undernourished would have been even lower than the present level.

Table   7.2

Percentage of income occurring to households in each decile

Declies	1973-74	1991-92
Lowest 5%	1.2	1.0
Decile 1	2.8	2.6
2	4.2	3.9
3	5.4	5.0
4	5.9	5.9
5	7.1	7.1
6	8.0	8.4
7	10.0	10.1
8	12.8	12.1
9	16.0	15.6
10	28.4	29.2
Top 5%	16.4	18.9

Source: BBS Household Expenditure Surveys
1991-92 and 1973-74

Further support for decline in hunger and undernutrition in Bangladesh is provided by demographic data. Undernutrition has many negative effects on a human population, of which death is the most serious. Although death due to undernutrition is not uncommon among adults, it is most visible among infants and children. Diarrhoea, cholera, pneumonia, bronchitis, marasmus, and koshiorkar are the most common killers. These diseases account for 40 percent of childhood deaths in Third World countries. In the opinion of one nutrition expert, 57 percent of infant deaths in Third World countries are due to undernutrition (Bengoa 1972). Thus, infant mortality rates are good indicators of nutritional status. High infant mortality represents widespread undernutrition.

In Bangladesh, infant mortality has consistently declined during the two decades.

156

During the reference period, it declined very substantially (Table 7.3). In 1992, it was 31 percent lower that in 1972. Therefore, demographic data also provide overwhelming evidence that hunger and undernutrition in Bangladesh have declined very significantly. Hence, our analysis based on HES, food production, per capita availability, and demographic data provide no support for those who have expressed strong doubts about the decline of hunger and undernutrition in Bangladesh (Ravallian 1990, Osmani 1991). Both writers strongly criticised differences in methodology employed for estimating undernutrition and data collection, but made no effort to seek support or lack of it from other indicators of undernutrition.

Table   7.3
Infant mortality rates per 1000 live births

Years	Both sexes
1974	1537
1975	138
1976	103
1977	114
	1974-77 average = 127
1980	102
1981	112
1982	122
1983	118
1984	122
1985	112
1986	117
1987	113
1988	116
1989	98
1990	94
1991	92
1992	88
	1989-92 average = 93

Source: BBS Statistical Yearbooks, various issues

Regional concentration of hunger

It is unfortunate that regional concentration of hunger in Bangladesh cannot be precisely identified, because household expenditure and actual food consumption are both reported only at the national scale. However, some knowledge about regional concentration of hunger can be gained from the identification of food surplus and deficit regions. Presumably, there will be a greater concentration of hunger and undernutrition in the food deficit regions, because in deficit regions a complex combination of some variables make food difficult to obtained for low income earners. First, food prices in deficit regions are relatively high because demand is greater than supply, and therefore a higher household income will be required to meet MRDCR. Second, because of low production there is less work, leading to fewer income earning opportunities, especially in rural areas. Because there is less demand for labour, employers tend to take advantage of the situation and depress wage. Hence, in food deficit regions, higher food prices and low incomes make it more difficult for the poor to acquire sufficient food for all members of the household. Some households, whose food intake would have been above the MRDCR, if living in a food surplus region, are pushed down below the MRDCR level in deficit regions.

In food surplus regions, on the other hand, larger volume of production creates more work for agricultural labourers, artisans, porters, transport workers, retailers, and a host of other workers. Besides more income earning opportunities, food prices in surplus regions will be relatively lower, because supply is greater than demand. Furthermore, greater demand for labour will improve the bargaining power of labour, who will push wages up. Therefore, households, who might have been below the MRDCR in a deficit region may have a good chance of being above MRDCR in a surplus region.

Food surplus and deficit regions

The BBS was publishing food surplus and deficit data by districts and *Upzilas* (the smallest statistical unit in Bangladesh, previously called *thana*) until 1982-83, but after that year, for some reason, they stopped publishing such data.

For measuring food surplus or deficit one has to determine net food supply and compare it with requirements in each region. The BBS measured supply only in terms of rice and wheat output. They deflated the output by 10 percent to allow for the proportion of output given to stock, kept for seed, and wasted during storage and transportation. They calculated the requirement for the total population, at the rate of 15.4 oz of cereals per head. This method apparently has some serious weaknesses. First, rice and wheat account for only 59 percent of the food quantity consumed per head or 78 percent of the calories in the average diet. Second, BBS does not seem to take into account the age and sex structure of the population in calculating food requirements, which appears statistically rather crude (BBS 1985).

I have measured food surplus and deficit more precisely for Bangladesh and each of its districts. The measurement is based on the ten most important food items in the average diet of a Bangladeshi, which include not only cereals but also pulses, fruits and vegetables, and fish. The ten most important items are rice, wheat, masur, grams, potatoes, brinjals, banana, mango, jackfruit, and fish. These account for 90 percent of the quantity of the average diet. The inclusion of pulses, fruits, vegetables, and fish is justified because large quantities of these are produced in the

158

country, and significant quantities of these are included even in the diet of the very poor. Some fruits and vegetables are cheaper than cereals when in season. Occasionally, poor households substitute them for cereals. For example, when potatoes, brinjals, and other vegetables are very cheap, the poor cook them with rice, in order to save some rice for the next meal. Similarly, the poor get considerable calories and other nutrients from seasonal fruits, which they may get from the trees around their own dwellings or may be given free by neighbours. The poor may even buy some over-ripe fruits from the market at very low prices. Sometimes, they may even be allowed to collect them free because they are not good enough for sale. Similarly, even fish is commonly used in the average diet, although infrequently by the poor.

To minimize annual fluctuations in food supply, I took a three year average (1989-90 to 1991-92) of each food item. Using the same deflator as used by BBS and others, the average output of each item was deflated by 10 percent, to get the net supply (BBS 1985, ICMR 1951). The supply of each item was then converted into calories. The sum of calories obtained from the 10 items gave the net food supply. I converted the total population into consumer units for the purpose of calculating food requirement. For this purpose, I multiplied the total population by 0.773 - a coefficient developed by Singh and applied by several researchers, which takes into account the age and sex of the population for food consumption purposes (Singh 1947, Census of India 1951, Chakravarti 1970). Finally, the net supply of calories was divided by the number of consumer units in each district to get per capita calorie supply. The districts, where the daily per capita supply was more then 2,122, were considered surplus, and where it was less than that, were considered deficit.

The average food supply in Bangladesh, obtained from the ten selected food items, was sufficient to provide 2035 calories per day to each consumer unit, which was 96 percent of the MRDCR level used by BBS to identify hunger and undernutrition. Some researchers would consider 2035 calories per person per day as sufficient nourishment (Ahmad, Khan, and Sampath 1991). In 1991-92, if we take only one year's production, the net food supply was sufficient to provide 2,132 calories per day to each consumer unit. Since food production in Bangladesh has been consistently increasing, it may be quite right to say that Bangladesh achieved self sufficiency in 1992. Even if we take a three year average food supply, the shortage is very small, and will be easily wiped out if one includes other food items such as oil, meat, sugar, and other fruits and vegetables in calculating food supply. Hence, domestic food supply is large enough to completely eradicate hunger and undernutrition, if equally distributed. But equal distribution is never possible, either in Bangladesh or anywhere else. So the problem of hunger and undernutrition in Bangladesh, at present, is not of inadequate supply but of distribution, as in most other countries of the world - developed and less developed. This brings out the essential difference between the food balance sheets and HES. If we look at the total food supply and requirements, we get the impression that there has been no hunger and undernutrition in Bangladesh at least in 1992, but the HES of 1991-92, which looks at the food consumption patterns in individual households, reveals that the food intake of about 47 percent of the population is still below the MRDCR.

The average per capita daily intake of calories in 1991-92 was 2,132- 7 percent above the MRDCR for Bangladesh - yet close to half the population was undernourished in the same year. Obviously, such a situation reveals that some members of the community were consuming a lot more than MRDCR. Ironically, people in higher income groups, who often have sedentary occupations and therefore don't need more than MRDCR, invariably consume more than the recommended allowance. The per capita expenditure on food for the three highest income groups is 137 percent higher than for the three lowest income groups. In terms of quantity too, the per capita consumption of food in the three highest income groups is 1.8 times more than in the three lowest income groups. Since the quantity of cereals consumed is about the same for both the groups, people in the higher income groups must be consuming much larger quantities of high calorie food. For example, they consume 12 times more meat and poultry and 2.5 times more fish. Such a consumption pattern is not unique to Bangladesh, but is common almost everywhere. People in higher income groups invariably consume more calories than they need and suffer from overnutrition.

The regional picture reveals large deviations from the national average in surplus and deficit. At the two extreme ends of the scale are Bogra and Dhaka. The net food supply for Bogra was 87 percent above the requirement, and that of Dhaka 57 percent below. Of the 20 districts, ten are food surplus and ten food deficit (Table 7.4).

The food surplus districts form a large contiguous area occupying much of the north and northwestern part of the country. Sylhet, Mymensingh (including Kishoreganj), Jamaplur, Bogra, Rangpur, Dinajpur, and Rajshahi comprise the contiguous food surplus region in the north and northwest. Three more surplus districts, namely, Jessore, Patuakhali, and Chittagong H.T. are outside the contiguous band. The surplus production is largely in the less densely populated districts, where there is also a marked concentration of irrigation. In 7 out of 10 food surplus districts, the percentage of TCA irrigated is greater than the national average, and with only one exception the irrigated area increased between 1973-74 and 1991-92.

The food deficit districts occupy central and coastal locations, largely in the lower section of the delta. They have fertile soils, good soil moisture, high population density, a marked concentration of small agricultural holdings, and a high percentage of population in agriculture, with a few exceptions. It appears that large agricultural population works hard on the small holdings to make a living, but with little success. Despite high input of labour, they are not able to produce enough to meet the MRDCR. Further, their efforts to produce enough food are marred by more than normal damage to crops by natural disasters, due to their locations. For example, in Comilla, Noakhali, Faridpur, Mymensingh, and Pabna, the crop damage due to natural disasters is much higher than the national average. Therefore, part of the problem in several food deficit districts is uncertainty of food supply. The largest deficiency occurs in the most urbanized districts, namely, Dhaka, Chittagong, and Khulna, largely because the density of total population on agricultural land is very high. Such regions are bound to be food deficit areas and must be supported from surplus production elsewhere within the country or imports from overseas.

Table 7.4
Food surplus and deficit regions, 1989-92 average

Districts	Per capita daily supply Calories	Surplus/deficit percent of MRDCR (2122 calories)	
Chittagong HT	2451	115.0	+
Chittagong	1489	70.2	-
Comilla	1336	62.9	-
Noakhali	1836	86.5	-
Sylhet	2227	105.0	+
Dhaka	890	42.0	-
Faridpur	1503	72.1	-
Jamalpur	2140	101.0	+
Mymensingh	2605	122.8	+
Tangil	1937	91.3	-
Barisal	1886	88.9	-
Jessore	3133	147.6	+
Khulna	1826	86.5	-
Kushtia	1987	93.6	-
Patuakhali	2834	133.6	+
Bogra	3962	186.7	+
Dinajpur	3424	161.4	+
Pabna	1724	81.2	-
Rajshahi	2559	120.6	+
Rangpur	2591	122.1	+
BANGLADESH	2035	95.9	-

Source: Calculated by the author from BBS data

It appears that in the densely populated food deficit districts, in the south and southeast, the maximum limit of increasing food production has been almost reached. Also, these districts are low lying and more prone to natural disasters, and therefore further investment in capital and labour for increasing food production may not be very rewarding. Attention should be directed more to the less populated surplus districts. Perhaps that is already happening, as we noted in Chapter 5.

Hunger and 'entitlement failure' in Bangladesh

Sen's theory of 'exchange entitlement' appears suitable for providing some explanation for hunger amidst plenty in Bangladesh (Sen 1981). One's entitlement to food is determined by what one has that can be exchanged for food in the market. The majority of those who are undernourished often only have their own labour power to exchange for food. Therefore, the quantity of food and other goods and services that they can buy depends on the market value of their labour power, i.e., the money value of labour wages relative to food and other goods. In other words, the quantity of food a labourer can buy depends on the exchange power of wage income. If wages do not increase in the same proportion as the price of food and other goods, the 'exchange entitlement' of labour is eroded. In this case, those at the lower end of the wage ladder will be forced to curtail the consumption of several goods and services, and some, who were adequately fed before, will be relegated to the undernourished category.

The erosion of 'exchange entitlement' is commonly initiated by a drop in supply. In the case of food, the drop in supply may be caused by partial crop failure, or a drop in food imports due to inadequate foreign exchange earnings. A drop in food supply is followed by a rise in food prices, a drop in demand for labour, and consequently a drop in wages. Therefore food becomes relatively more expensive. Whenever there is a drop in food supply, those who do not own any land or very little of it are most affected, those who produce their own food and have a surplus are least affected.

Sometimes the 'exchange entitlement' may be eroded without any drop in supply. This happens when food prices rise due to hoarding, exports, or increased consumption by some relatively more prosperous sections of the community. Under such circumstances, there will be no increase in wages, because there is no increase in the demand for labour as production remains unchanged. Hence, erosion of 'exchange entitlement' is possible without any drop in supply.

In Bangladesh, as we have already seen, the total food supply and also per capita supply both increased between 1972-73 and 1991-92. The increased supply and its multiplier effects considerably reduced hunger and undernutrition. This gives the impression that during this period the 'exchange entitlement' of labour must have improved and contributed to the reduction of hunger. The 'exchange entitlement' of labour indeed increased during the period, but not consistently. Between 1970-71 and 1983-84, agricultural labourers, who form the most vulnerable section of the society, experienced an erosion of their entitlement (Dayal 1988). During this period, the money value of wages in Bangladesh agriculture did not keep pace with the cost of food normally consumed by labourers. The cost of the standard daily diet of an agricultural labourer increased 641 percent, but money wages only 493 percent. Hence an agricultural labourer and his dependents were worse off in 1983-84 in terms of nutritional intake compared with the base year (Figure 7.1). The gap

162

between money wages and the cost of the standard daily diet was clearly increasing throughout the period. It was at its maximum in 1974-75, the famine year. This situation arose because food prices rose steeply between 1973-74 and 1974-75, but money wages maintained the average growth rate that prevailed over the previous three years (Sen 1981, Dayal 1988). After the famine year (1974-75) food prices began to drop as sharply as they had previously risen, but money wages remained stable at the 1974-75 level for the next three years. Overall, between 1974-75 and 1975-76 food prices dropped by 32 percent. This is an interesting observation and seems to provide support for the classical theory of wages. In the light of the subsistence theory of wages, two possible explanations can be given for the negative response of wages to declining food prices during the three years following famine.

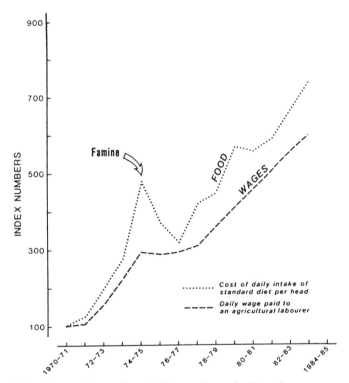

Figure 7.1 Cost of standard diet and agricultural wages over time
Source: E. Dayal, Canadian Geographer, 1988

First, employers have a vested interested in maintaining the physical strength of labour, to a certain level at least, as it directly affects work capacity and, consequently, productivity. The level of nutritional intake of agricultural workers in Bangladesh has always been very low, and so it was before the famine. During the famine and the following year the wages relative to food prices were too low to

163

provide enough nutrition to subsist. Hence, a further drop in nutritional intake would have harmed the general health and working capacity of labourers. Many workers, especially those who had many dependents to feed, must have become weak from a greatly reduced intake of food during the famine. This would have reduced productivity during the famine, which would have continued to decline if wages were lowered in accordance with the declining food prices. Employers therefore did not lower wages when food prices began to drop after the famine (1974-75), because they had a personal interest in rebuilding the physical strength and stamina of workers that were lost during the famine. In essence they took a medium rather that a short-term view of gains. They might, therefore, have allowed some time for the regaining of the lost strength of labourers.

Second, a higher mortality due to sickness and protein-calorie malnutrition during the famine might have depleted the labour supply during the famine. Hence, again, it was in the interest of the landlords to allow somewhat more than normal nutritional intake in order to rebuild the reduced labour supply. These two objective may have been part of the reason for not lowering wages to follow food prices after the famine for some years.

From 1976-77 food prices and wages began to rise again, but with the former rising faster than the latter. The cost of the standard diet and the value of money wages rose at the rate of 52.5 and 37.6 percent per year, respectively. Although the cost of the standard diet was rising faster than wages, even before the famine, the gap in the growth rates of the two was slightly smaller than after 1976-77 (Figure 7.1). This is attributable to the breaking down of the wage adjustment mechanism, which weakened the bargaining power of labour (Ravallion 1982). While a drop in labour supply should theoretically have led to a steeper rise in wages, in reality the weak and sick labour force was in no position to bargain. Some reduction in the gap between wages and food costs occurred between 1979-80 and 1981-82, but thereafter the gap began to widen again. Khan (1977) identified somewhat similar fluctuations in real wages during 1949-75.

The above analysis clearly demonstrates that the real value of wages was eroded over time in Bangladesh. In the initial year 1970-71, the nutritional wage (the number of calories that a wage could provide, from the most basic foods consumed by agricultural labourers) was 6,203 calories. It reached the lowest level, 3,843 calories, in 1974-75, 35 percent less than the 1970-71 value. It recovered slightly after the famine but never reached the 1970-71 level again. In 1983-84, the nutritional wage was only 80 percent of the 1970-71 level, or 1,235 calories below its nutritional value in the base year.

From the mid 1980s, food supply began to increase rapidly, despite the devastating floods of 1987 and 1988. The increased food supply through its many linkages began to substantially improve the economy and, consequently, the position of labour. Throughout the 1970s, the increase in food prices remained above wages, relative to 1972-73, but the difference was very small. Nevertheless, the trend indicates erosion of exchange entitlement of wages (Figure 7.2). It was only since 1981-82 that the relative increase in wages began to be higher than food prices, but, again, the difference was very small. It was only from 1985-86 that the relative increase in wages began to be very significantly higher than food prices. The relative increase in wages dropped again in 1987-88 to reach the level of food prices, presumably because of serious floods in those years. But after 1987-88, wages began to increase much faster than food prices, and the difference in favour of wages became larger than ever before. The 'exchange entitlements' of wages began to improve rapidly. The data for the early 1990s seem to show that this trend is going to continue (Figure 7.2).

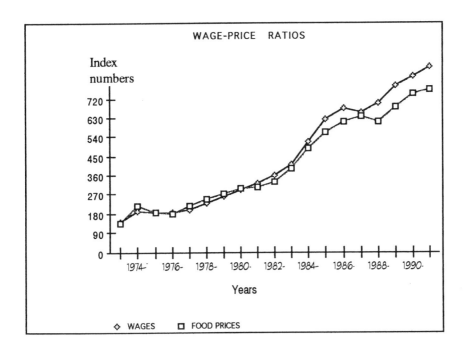

Figure 7.2   Food exchange ratios of agricultural wages

Over the period between 1973-74 and 1991-92, the entitlements improved considerably, as displayed by the income and expenditure data at constant and current prices for individuals and households. Between 1973-74 and 1991-92, the annual per capita income and expenditure at constant prices increased by 26 and 8 percent respectively (Table 7.5). The greater increase in income than expenditure was recorded at the national, urban, and rural levels. The lower increase in expenditure than income reflects a slower rise in the cost of food and other goods. If the cost had increased in the same proportion as income, the expenditure also would have increased in the same proportion. Also, monthly consumption expenditure indicates a very significant proportional decline in expenditure on food. Between 1973-74 and 1991-92, the consumption expenditure on food dropped from 74.2 to 66.6 percent of

165

the total consumption expenditure. Hence, changes in income, total expenditure, and proportion of consumption expenditure on food all indicate that there has been a general increase in entitlements.

Table   7.5
Annual per capita income and expenditure at constant 1991-92 prices in Takas

	1973-74	1991-92	Percentage change
Income	4,920	6,205	26.1
Expenditure	5,199	5,615	8.0

Source: Calculated by the author from BBS data

The changes in income and expenditure in rural and urban areas both show that urban bias in development is continuing. The levels of per capita and household incomes as well as expenditure and their increases are much higher in the urban areas. The urban incomes in the final year were 158 percent of rural incomes, compared with 135 percent in the base year. The difference is clearly increasing in favour of urban areas.

As seen in a previous section, erosion of exchange entitlement of agricultural wages and therefore labour power, occurred during the 1970s and early 1980s, and the prospects of reducing hunger appeared dismal during those years. But fortunately the 'entitlement failure' was arrested in the mid 1980s. The improvement of entitlements enabled people to eat better and rise above the level of undernutrition. The most obvious reason for improvements in entitlements from the mid 1980s and drop in hunger appears to be a very substantial rise in food supply. The increased supply probably had a depressing effect on food prices. They continued to increase even after the mid 1980s, but not as steeply as in the 1970s. Further, the multiplier effects of increasing supply created more income-earning opportunities, greater demand for labour at higher wages. All available indicators seem to show that this trend is very likely to continue into the 1990s.

Factors affecting hunger

Despite inadequate data and many conceptual issues still unresolved, several studies have been focused on the measurement of hunger, its change over time, and the variables affecting it (Ahluwalia 1978 and 1985, Bardhan 1973, Dandekar and Rath

166

1971, Dandekar 1981, Sukhatme 1982, Mellor and Desai 1985, BDS 1990). Much of the debate initially was centred on analyzing poverty trends. Later, attention was directed to variables affecting hunger, particularly agricultural performance and food prices. In Bangladesh, the main thrust of hunger studies has been on the analysis of trends in hunger and undernutrition, and no attempt, to my knowledge, has been made to identify the factors affecting it. Therefore, this section is concerned with the identification of variables that have contributed to reduction of hunger in the country. I have employed a multiple regression model for the purpose:

$$Y = a + b_1X_1 + b_2X_2 \quad \dots\dots\dots\dots\dots\dots\dots\dots \quad (1)$$

where Y = the extent of hunger (percent of population consuming less then the recommended calories)

X_1 = net per capita availability of foodgrains including minor cereals

X_2 = food exchange ratio of agricultural wages (food purchasing power of wages)

The two independent variables were chosen because they capture the effect of the four most important factors affecting hunger. The extent of hunger in any region may be affected by the size of the food supply, the size of the consuming population, wages, and food prices. In equation (1), X_1 - net per capita availability of foodgrains captures the effect of food supply and the consuming population. X_2, food exchange ratio (kilograms of rice an agricultural wage can buy), which represents the exchange entitlement of agricultural workers, captures the effect of wages and food prices on hunger. Another variable which exerts an important influence on hunger is distribution of income, but that could not be included in this model.

The data for all three variables was obtained from BBS. Nineteen-year time series, from 1973-74 to 1991-92, were formed for X_1 and X_2. Y values were available only for six HES years. Since the percentage of hungry in Bangladesh has been consistently declining, the missing values were obtained by interpolation techniques.

The inter-correlation between the two explanatory variables is only modest at r = 0.63, and therefore is not expected to distort the results very much. As there is no a priori basis for predicting the exact form of a regression model, first, a linear form was employed. It produced highly significant results and gave no indication that a transformation would improve results. Although, in a previous section, I made some speculations about the variables that may affect the extent of hunger, this section seeks statistical support for the speculations.

The model (1) is statistically highly significant and explains 80 percent of the variation in hunger over time (Table 7.6). Both coefficients for the explanatory variables are, as expected, negative and highly significant, indicating that both per capita availability of food and exchange entitlement of wages have a profound

167

influence on hunger. We have already noted earlier that exchange entitlement of wages began to increase from the mid 1980s. In 1988, food prices declined but wages continued to increase, resulting in a very significant improvement in exchange entitlements. The inverse relationship between hunger on the one hand, and food supply and exchange entitlement on the other, confirm the views expressed earlier and provide empirical support for Sen's theory of 'exchange entitlement'. The regression results show that although exchange entitlement exerts a very profound influence on hunger, food supply is also important. This relationship was also noted by Jain in his review of poverty alleviation programs in India (Jain 1986). He argued that increasing purchasing power alone without a parallel increase in production (food supply) was not going to improve food intake.

Table 7.6
Regression results: variables affecting change in hunger

Explanatory variables	Regression coefficients	t-ratios
Per capita availability of foodgrains	-0.613[a]	-2.67
Food exchange ratio of agricultural wages	- 14.559[b]	- 4.71
Constant	208.79[b]	5.92
R^2=82.4[b]		
F=37.44[b]		
N=20		

Note : a Significant at .01 level
         b Significant at .001 level

The positive correlation between X_1 and X_2 indicates that a rise in food supply improves exchange entitlement. This means that the higher the supply the better the exchange ratio of wages. Therefore, a rise in the two variables together tends to lower the level of hunger. In Bangladesh, because wages and prices are largely determined by market forces, it follows that in a free economy food supply through its various linkages exerts a very important influence on the extent of hunger. Therefore, government policy to increase food supply through increased application of irrigation and other modern inputs is in the right direction. Since exchange entitlement of wages is quite independent of production data and HES expenditure data, the results of the regression model prove a very important point, that a

168

reduction in hunger and undernutrition in the 1980s was very real. It was certainly not a 'statistical illusion' as described by Osmani (1990).

Summary

To identify the undernourished, Bangladesh employs an MRDCR level of 2,122 calories per consumption unit, developed by FAO/WHO for South Asia. Based on the above level, the analysis in this chapter reveals that hunger in Bangladesh has declined considerably during the two decades. Between the first and the last HESs, conducted in 1973-74 and 1991-92, the proportion of undernourished dropped from 83 to 47 percent of the total population. This conclusion is well supported by a decline in infant mortality and changes in other demographic variables and an increase in the domestic food supply during the same period. In 1991-92, the domestic food supply, obtained from 10 selected food items, was sufficient to provide 2,132 calories to each consumer unit, which was 7 percent above the MRDCR. The increase in income inequality during the period was too small to alter the above conclusion.

Hunger in Bangladesh appears to be more concentrated in the densely populated and food deficit central and coastal districts.

During the two decades, the food exchange entitlements of individuals increased considerably, as displayed by the income and expenditure data at constant prices and food exchange rates of agricultural wages. The regression model used in this chapter indicates that per capita availability of food and the food exchange ratio of wages are important variables affecting the extent of hunger. Together they account for 80 percent of the variation in the extent of hunger over time.

8 Hunger alleviation

The two most important requirements for the alleviation of hunger are increasing food supply and the purchasing power of the poor. Mellor (1988) has forcefully argued that increasing food production is essential for hunger eradication. Sen (1981) also recognizes the importance of food availability and output in increasing food entitlement or in hunger reduction, but he argues that increased output does not automatically increase the food entitlement of all. Increased production may increase the food entitlement of those who are producing their own food but are at the margin of hunger. For example, small farmers, who may suffer from partial hunger in normal years, may move out of hunger in a good year because their food output might have increased sufficiently to meet their requirements. The link between food availability and food entitlement is complex. The actual command over food is determined not only by availability but a set of complex legal and economic variables, among which food purchasing power is the most important. Increased availability of food increases food entitlement through employment creation for those who are involved in actual production but they (agricultural labourers) do not have a legal right on increased production (Dreze and Sen 1989). There is considerable evidence that increased food supply also has a positive impact on individual incomes (Jain 1986, Khan 1990, Subramanian 1975). Khan (1990) has provided quantitative evidence that cereal production in Bangladesh is positively related to GNP and negatively to the retail price of rice. The linkages between production and individual incomes have already been discussed in the previous chapter. There appears to be general agreement that increasing food supply is an essential ingredient in the recipe for hunger alleviation (Dreze and Sen 1989, Gillespie and Neill 1992). As the trends in food supply have already been examined in some detail in Chapter 4, the focus in this chapter will be on the role of the government in increasing food supply and protecting the purchasing power of the poor in Bangladesh since independence.

Domestic food supply and the state

The government in Bangladesh is committed to achieving self-sufficiency in food supply and reducing hunger, and in this venture it has received much assistance from several developed countries, particularly the USA, and several international organizations. Historically, the domestic private sector has made little contribution to the development of the rural infrastructure that is required for increasing food supply. This is because the return on capital investment in building roads, bridges, and irrigation network is low and the capital requirement is large, often beyond the capacity of private individuals. Also, most farms are small and widely scattered, making investment in agricultural and rural development less attractive. However, in the Third Five Year Plan (1985-1990), the private sector investment in agricultural development was about half the investment by the public sector. This probably happened when HYRVs had spread over a considerable area, and clearly demonstrated that investment in new rice technology was very profitable. The private sector then began to invest in fertilizers, insecticides, irrigation equipment, and minor irrigation such as shallow tube wells that yield short-term benefits. However, the private sector did not make any significant investment in infrastructure facilities that have long-term benefits.

Development of rural infrastructure and institutions

Realizing that initially the irrigation facilities in the country were entirely inadequate for agricultural development, particularly for promoting HYRVs, the government set up the Bangladesh Water Development Board (BWDB) and the Bangladesh Agricultural Development Corporation (BADC), which were made responsible for the development of water resources. Although both institutions were responsible for developing water resources, they were assigned special functions. While BWDB was entrusted with the development of large-scale irrigation, drainage, and flood control, the BADC, among other things, was given the responsibility of developing minor irrigation projects - low collect pumps and deep and shallow tube wells. Besides the development of water resources, BADC was also given responsibility for the procurement of fertilizers and HYV seeds. The government also realized that provision of inputs alone was not going to be very effective in increasing food production because of the deplorable conditions that prevailed in rural areas. The rural areas of Bangladesh were grossly neglected not only during the British colonial period but also during the Pakistani regime. The economic underdevelopment was marked by concentration of poverty, landlessness, unemployment, and low productivity in rural areas. Further, there was also a severe dearth of 'infrastructural facilities' such as roads, drainage, markets, and social services like health, education, and sanitation. The government, therefore, assumed responsibility for the development of infrastructure in the rural areas because it was essential for increasing food supply.

Further, the rural areas in Bangladesh suffered from serious lack of administrative institutions. The Moguls and, after them, the British colonial authorities neglected rural areas and exercised control over them only indirectly through indigenous landholders, called *zamindars*, who were revenue collectors and keepers of the peace. The rural areas became "rural hinterland simply to serve distant urban centres within the sub-continent and the more distant metropoles overseas" (Johnson 1974). The city-based merchants bought exportable items in periodic markets from a large number of small rural producers, who were in desperate need of some cash income. The city-based merchants had working capital and the backing of commercial banks. The buyers were few in number as against a multitude of small producers in rural periodic markets. The buyers exploited the situation and bought the items at the lowest possible prices. The multitude of sellers performed some important functions such as collection, transport, and grading of products at a very low cost. The city-based merchants were quite happy with this arrangement and had no economic reason to change it. This pattern of trade is often called 'vertical trade' and is believed to have developed during the colonial period (Johnson 1974). It prevented the development of 'horizontal trade' between market centres. The flow of goods is only in one direction, i.e., from rural markets to the colonial city. Hence, it did not expose the rural producers to the urban market economy. The impact of vertical trade on the rural community is well described by Johnson,"This trade does nothing to integrate town and country, nor does it promise to make any contribution to the development of more complex, differentiated, and efficient rural economic centres" (Johnson 1974, p. 88). This legacy of pre-colonial and colonial times has continued to retard development of rural areas into the present. It initiated the concentration of hunger and poverty in rural areas by a variety of policies. The colonial policies discouraged handicraft industries and food crop production. The colonial authorities encouraged and sometimes forced the cultivation of cash crops such as indigo, jute, tobacco, and sugarcane. The authorities occupied the best land for indigo cultivation, and also forced local farmers — by first giving them loans — to cultivate idigo for them. Ryot (1858) strongly felt that indigo cultivation in Bengal was oppressive and cruel.

For increasing food supply and employment opportunities in rural areas, where hunger and poverty are concentrated, there was a desperate need for making a variety of improvements for uplifting the rural community so that they could participate in and benefit from modern agricultural technologies. In order to create a healthy and at least moderately informed community, it was necessary to improve health, sanitation, education, and accessibility in rural areas. There is ample evidence that the government of independent Bangladesh has made considerable investment to improve these areas, and to make rural areas suitable for increasing food supply.

Besides organizing the supply of modern inputs, there was an urgent need for introducing agricultural support programs in order to take modern technology to the farmer and thus reduce the gap between the technocrats and the users. It was also necessary to raise the level of literacy and general education in rural areas so that farmers could comprehend the benefits of modern technology and avoid its disadvantages. For example, some education is required to know the disadvantages of excessive use of fertilizers, insecticides, pesticides, machinery, and even irrigation. "The expansion of universal primary education was recognised as the cornerstone of development of human resources" (Planning Commission, 1983, p. 97). The government launched a scheme for the promotion and expansion of agricultural education at all levels, particularly at the *thana* and village levels. Besides research organizations such as the Bangladesh Rice Research Institute (BRRI), the BADC, the Bangladesh Agricultural Research Institute (BARI) at the national level, and agricultural universities at the regional level, a large number of extension and training centres were opened at the *thana* and village levels to train personnel at the sub-technical levels. In order to make best use of local resources, extension workers visit farming activities on a regular basis. They advise and supervise the activities of farmers. This has narrowed the gap between research and practice.

Rapid expansion of modern agricultural technology required expansion of agricultural research facilities and training of research personnel. The public sector played an important role in this area by establishing several research organizations such as the Bangladesh Agricultural Research Council (BARC), (BWDB), BARI, BRRI, BADC, and the National Seed Board (NSB). The research organizations have made notable contributions to the improvement and diversification of the crop pattern, soil and water management, increased crop yields, and food supply.

The government's commitment to reduction of hunger and poverty in Bangladesh is also clearly reflected in the allocation of funds in the development plans. In all development plans, the objective of increasing food supply received a high priority; it was an important part of the basic development philosophy. To improve living standards by ensuring adequate supply of basic needs has been a major objective of development planning. About a third of the total outlay in the first four plans was allocated to the development of agriculture and the rural community (Table 8.1).

Table 8.1

Allocation of development funds to agriculture, irrigation, and rural development during successive development plans

	Percentage of total plans allocation
First Plan (1973-78)	31.2
Two Year Plan (1978-80)	28.9
Second Plan	29.1
Third Plan (1986-90)	28.0
Fourth Plan	26.0

Source: Compiled by the author from BBS data

Agricultural development included the development of water resources, i.e., minor and major irrigation projects, drainage, and flood control. It also included provision of facilities required for the promotion of HYRVs, i.e., production and distribution of fertilizers, insecticides, credit facilities and HYV seeds. The government of independent Bangladesh realized quite early that, without rapid promotion of HYRVs, self-sufficiency in food supply could not be achieved. Prior to independence, not much was done to promote agricultural development in the region which is now Bangladesh. A quick glance at the data for the use of modern inputs in agriculture displays how badly the agricultural sector was neglected in Bangladesh when it was under Pakistan (Table 8.2, Hossain 1984). For example, the area under HYRVs in 1969-70 was a mere 2.1 percent of the TCA, but within 6 years after independence it jumped to 13 percent. More than half the cropped area in rice is now under HYRVs. A similar picture is portrayed by data for irrigation and fertilizer use (Table 8.2). The percentage of the cultivated area irrigated by modern methods increased by 18 percentage points, and fertilizer consumption more than quadrupled between 1970 and 1992. The promotion of water-fertilizer-seed technology has made the biggest contribution to the achievement of near self-sufficiency in food supply and to hunger reduction. The infrastructure for the spread of HYV seeds initially was almost entirely provided by the public sector, because farmers would not make investment in irrigation and drainage. The rapid expansion of HYVs created a large demand for modern inputs and much bigger distribution machinery than provided by

Table 8.2
Use of modern inputs in agriculture over time

Years	Area irrigated by modern methods as a percent of cultivated land	HYV area as percent of cultivated land	Fertilizers lbs per cropped acre
1960-61	0.3	nil	2
1965-66	0.9	nil	4
1969-70	2.6	2.1	9
1975-76	7.7	13.0	15
1979-80	12.8	18.6	28
1982-83	19.2	22.9	31
1990-91*	27.0	47.4	206

Source: Adapted from Hossain 1984. * Computed from BBS data

BADC. Therefore, the services provided by BADC became inefficient and also corrupt (Hossain and Jones 1983). Similarly, as the volume of fertilizers used increased, the government expenditure on subsidies also increased. At the end of the

1970s, the fertilizer subsidies consumed 25 percent of the agricultural development budget. The government was then pressurized to transfer the distribution of modern agricultural inputs to the private sector. Gradually, therefore, the distribution of fertilizers, insecticides, and irrigation equipment was successfully privatized. Now private dealers are paid a commission for collecting fertilizers and other inputs from primary distribution points and selling them to consumers. The primary distribution points are still managed by BADC.

When Bangladesh became independent, the views about development were changing. In the 1950s and 1960s, the emphasis was on economic growth. It was believed that the benefits of growth would eventually be passed on to the poor. This concept is known as the 'trickle down theory of development' in economic literature. In the late 1960s, it was realized that this was not happening. The rapid growth of the economy was making the rich richer and the poor poorer, consequently increasing the gap between the rich and the poor. Hence, poverty in the rural areas persisted. Prior to 1970s the central objective of rural development was to increase agricultural productivity and production. After the 1970s, the emphasis shifted from growth only to growth with justice. Reduction of poverty and also of inequality became important objectives in development planning, particularly in rural development. It was realized that large projects were not doing much to improve the lot of the poor. Small-scale projects in irrigation and other spheres of development began to receive priority. It was only in small scale projects that the poor could also participate in decision making and benefit more from them. On this count the government should be commended for making a right choice of technology in their development planning. They realized that one of the most valuable assets of the country was a large and cheap labour force that must be fully utilized for the benefit of all. Hence, they chose a technology that was advanced in some respects but labour intensive at the same time.

We have already seen that the private sector made little investment in the development of rural areas, and therefore the responsibility of developing rural areas fell on the government. The two most important programs for the improvement of rural areas initiated by the government in the early 1970s were the Integrated Rural Development Program (IRDP) and the Rural Works Programs (RWP). The concept of IRDP was not something new; it was first initiated by Mao and Gandhi (Lea and Chaudhri 1983). Both leaders felt that the key to poverty eradication lay in the villages. The IRDP envisaged not only increasing agricultural production but overall development of rural areas. It was concerned with uplifting the rural community and increasing the living standards of all. The main aim was to bring economic prosperity to all in rural areas and thereby reduce hunger and poverty. The program to develop rural institutions was first initiated by the East Pakistan government in the 1960s; later it was adopted by the Bangladesh Government and became known as IRDP. It was aimed at bringing government to local areas so that the local rural population could participate in decision making. The administrative machinery with centralized power at the district level was not well informed about the development problems at the 'grass roots', and had become inefficient in discharging its responsibility towards development. The establishment of a system of local government with power close to the rural problems was required for providing efficient support for agricultural development. Therefore, the government established several institutions at the local level to accelerate development. It established co-operative system of farmers (KSSS), *thana* training and development centres (TTDCs), the rural works program (RWP), and co-operative societies for landless rural population to create non-agricultural activities. By 1980, IRDP had spread to over 267 *thanas* out of the total of 475 *thanas*, and farmers co-operatives had jumped to 40,000 with a membership of 1.3 million (Hossain and Jones 1983). Nevertheless, the IRDP faces many problems of implementation. The groundwork required for effective implementation of the program was not properly done. Therefore, the selection of the target population is often not right, and sometimes it is even deliberately falsified. Often those who are in desperate need are by-passed as they cannot reach the right authorities because they are not influential. The rural elite, who are politically powerful, often influence the selection of households for the benefits of IRDP. The government lets the local elite interfere in the program to some extent in order to win their patronage. Thus, IRDP and other rural employment programs, despite their important contribution to rural development, also play an important political role for the government; they enhance their political authority (Sobhan 1990). Further, there is a long chain of intermediaries between the government and the poor, who are the target population of the IRDP. Therefore, by the time the benefits reach the poor, they are considerably reduced.

An important component of rural development is employment creation for the rural poor. About one-third of the rural households are landless and chronically unemployed. Less than half the heads of landless households can find seasonal jobs in agriculture. The rest of the landless households manage to exist by doing odd labouring jobs, such as cleaning toilets and drains, carting goods and people, skinning dead animals, and some are forced to beg. There are some who are artisans, such as carpenters, blacksmiths, barbers, and weavers, who may earn a reasonable income in good agricultural years, but normally they too do not get enough work to make a good living. They simply manage a meagre existence. If incomes of the rural poor do not rise, their continuance at a low level will be a serious impediment to agricultural development and the achievement of self-sufficiency in food supply. Low incomes of the poor will depress the effective demand and discourage surplus producers to increase production. The government is aware of this problem and has taken several positive steps to increase rural employment. It has launched two main rural works programs - RWP and the Food For Work Program (FFWP). The RWP and FFWP were aimed at creating new employment opportunities in rural areas. They were concerned with self-help projects, such as building roads, embankments, irrigation canals, dams, and drainage channels. The donors of development aid to Bangladesh supported the strategy of hunger alleviation through employment creation in small scale projects. Both programs are directed towards creating infrastructure needed for agricultural development, and have been successful in generating millions of man days of work for the rural unemployed. The physical achievements are also quite significant. Thousands of kilometres of roads, canals, and embankments have been constructed in rural areas through the two work programs. The technology used is deliberately labour-intensive, and it is believed to have a positive effect on productivity in the long run. Nevertheless, the achievements of the programs were marred by administrative inefficiency and corruption (Hossain and Jones 1983). Often the most needed projects were not given the highest priority, and those people most in need were not given work.

An important ingredient of rural and agricultural development, which only the government can initiate and implement, is land reform. I have already discussed the structure and distribution of agricultural holdings in Chapter 2. Here, I will only briefly discuss what the government has done in the area of land reform. Land reforms may include a variety of measures that may affect the manner in which land is owned, distributed, and used for cultivation. In Bangladesh, highly unequal distribution of land and its division into a large number of small and fragmented holdings is a major problem that holds back agricultural development. About 70 percent of the farm households own only 29 percent of the farm land, and only 10 percent of the large farm households own about 50 percent of the farm area (BBS 1986). Whether redistribution of land in a more equitable manner will increase agricultural production is debatable. One view is that redistribution will make a big difference because 98 percent of the landless rural households live in absolute poverty or are undernourished (Rahman 1985, Dixon 1990). In Bangladesh, landlessness is synonymous with hunger. I have already cited several studies in Chapter 5 that have concluded that productivity and intensity of cultivation are both high on small farms.

On the other hand, a second group of researchers believe that in Bangladesh there is simply not enough land in large farms. Therefore, a redistribution will not make much difference to landlessness or average farm size (Hossain 1977, Islam 1977, Hussain 1989). In their view, a redistribution is not likely to increase food supply and reduce food poverty. Even if redistribution is accepted as a policy by the government , several problems will arise in its implementation. First, to decide on an appropriate ceiling will be difficult. Second, in the extended family system that prevails in Bangladesh, it will be very difficult to implement any ceiling that may be decided upon. Nevertheless, despite these problems the government and also the opposition parties agreed in 1980 that some sort of land reforms for promoting growth and equity are desirable and must be discussed in the parliament. However, nothing seems to have been done. Using the land ceiling of 13.5 hectares that was introduced in 1971, only 0.3 percent of the cultivated area was declared surplus (Hossain and Jones 1983). Many large landowners, particularly in the western districts, continue to hold land much above 13.5 hectares. Some households divided the holding between the members of the extended family, and continued to hold land above the ceiling probably by bribing the local land revenue officers. Land reform measures have not been seriously undertaken because national politicians and bureaucrats are themselves big land owners. Further, the poor who are landless labourers and small cultivators depend so heavily on the big landlords that they

177

cannot form protest groups against the landlords or report any illegal practices the landlords may be involved in.

It may be concluded that any increase in food supply has to come without any major land reforms. Perhaps legislation focused on improving terms and conditions of tenancies will be more effective than land redistribution. The tenancy reforms will also not be liked by the big landowners but they may be more acceptable than land reforms.

The above discussion shows that the government in Bangladesh is genuinely interested in increasing domestic food production and reducing hunger in the country, and to achieve that it has taken action in several directions. The government has provided basic facilities for increasing agricultural production such as irrigation, flood control, drainage, distribution of inputs, credit, agricultural education and research, and rural employment. Further, it is essential to maintain an economic climate which gives an adequate return to the farmers on their investments (Chakravarti 1984). The government guarantees an adequate return by paying a fair procurement price, which has certainly raised growers' prices (Chowdhury 1987). The procurement system provides much needed incentives to the farmers to produce more. Because domestic production was not likely to meet requirements fully, it had to be supplemented with food obtained from outside. In this area too the government had an important role to play because the national economy is not based on free trade. Both imports and food aid are negotiated at the government to government level in Bangladesh. Therefore, in the next section of this chapter, we will examine the role of the government in obtaining food supply from outside the country.

The role of the state in procuring food from overseas

Because the domestic supply of food falls short of requirements, the government has to arrange imports of food from the world market, and also negotiate food aid from surplus countries and the WFP. The government tries to get food as outright grants, but often it has to agree to take food aid loans.

Food imports

Since its inception, Bangladesh has been a food deficit country. Between 10 to 12 percent of its food requirements came from outside in the form of food imports or aid throughout the 1970s and early 1980s. Although the magnitude of imports does not represent a great deal of dependence compared with most European countries, it drains away a big portion of country's meagre foreign exchange income, which includes export earnings and food and development aid from foreign donors. Bangladesh desperately needs hard currency for importing capital goods for development of the non-agricultural sector of the economy. Several countries in Europe, Southwest Asia, East Asia, and Latin America are much more dependent on food imports than Bangladesh, but the difference is that they have financial resources

178

to easily pay for food imports. However, it is very comforting to note that food imports in Bangladesh have declined very considerably in recent years. For example, between 1972 and 1992, imports of cereals and rice declined by 29 and 73 percent respectively. In 1972, rice imports were 5 percent of the domestic production, but in 1992 they were only 0.5 percent. The domestic production is now able to nearly meet the effective demand. Most of the food imports in Bangladesh have been paid for by foreign aid, and the magnitude of foreign aid depends on the extent to which the government can negotiate with other countries and organizations and on the political policies it pursues. Since the 1974 famine, the government has been successful in acquiring enough food from outside to supplement the domestic production and in avoiding acute food shortages.

Bangladesh has always suffered from a chronic balance of payment problem. It would have been very difficult for Bangladesh to pay for food imports without the large foreign aid that it gets. But no country can continue to depend on charity for food indefinitely. Therefore, it was essential for Bangladesh to achieve self-sufficiency sooner or later.

Bangladesh is continuing to import about 1.5 million metric tons of cereals annually, mostly wheat. This is largely to meet the increasing urban demand for western style bread and confectionery, which is due to a faster increase of the urban population and urban incomes than the national averages. The domestic production of wheat has been adversely affected by a rapid increase in winter rice. In 1992, 37 percent of rice production came from the winter rice crop, whereas in 1972 only 18 percent of rice came from winter rice. The government policy stresses expansion of winter rice, because it involves less risk from natural hazards. Therefore farmers are more willing to invest in inputs required for HYRVs in winter. *Boro* rice that is cultivated in winter competes with wheat. In the competition for a share of the cropland, rice wins because it is a more valuable crop and is in greater demand. Therefore, domestic production of wheat in recent years has been declining, after reaching a peak in the mid 1980s.

The growth of population and incomes in Bangladesh will continue to increase the demand for food, and therefore the need to import food may continue for sometime. Even when population and incomes are stabilized, imports of food will be required whenever there is widespread crop failure owing to natural hazards. Building large reserves of food in a damp climate with a high frequency of natural hazards would not only be difficult but also unsafe.

Food aid

Soon after Bangladesh became independent, food production costs and therefore food prices rose rapidly because of a steep rise in oil prices. Importing food for developing countries became very difficult and much more so for Bangladesh, because the domestic supply of food and, in fact, the whole economy had been badly disturbed during the war of liberation. However, Bangladesh had no choice but to import more food. Bangladesh had no resources to pay for food imports, and without foreign aid many thousands and perhaps millions of people might have died of starvation. During the two decades ending in 1992, Bangladesh received large volume of food aid largely from the USA, Canada, and Australia. All food aid that comes from these countries is in wheat. Australian food aid is given as an outright grant. In emergency situations, Australia also pays freight (ADAB 1983). Bangladesh is on the top of the list of countries that receive food aid from Australia. The volume of food aid to Bangladesh varies according to need, ie., the gap between domestic production and requirement in a given year. The main objectives of Australian aid are two-fold: one, to provide food for humanitarian relief of the poorer groups; and second, to contribute foodgrains for supporting the government's PFDS. About 30 percent of the food aid goes to support FFWP, and the remaining 70 percent goes to other components of the PFDS. The money earned from the sale of the foodgrains supplied as food aid must be used for developmental activities. The food aid given by the USA and Canada is much larger in volume, but it has more political strings attached to it. For example, the US food aid does not go to its communist political opponents such as Cuba, and even to the countries that trade with Cuba (Thomson 1992).

Initially, food aid was designed to sell surplus food from donor countries to needy developing countries on a variety of concessionary terms. Food aid helped Bangladesh in its development programs and in achieving near self-sufficiency. It has helped immensely in times of acute food scarcity caused by natural disasters. It has also helped the government to build reserve stocks, to provide employment to the poor, and to develop rural areas. But food aid has been strongly criticised for its direction and its effects on domestic production. Because of political strings attached to it, food aid often does not reach where it is most needed. It has also been noticed that food aid tends to depress local food prices, which is a disincentive to the local producers. Some have argued that food aid makes nations too dependent on others for their food supply and deters them from making serious efforts to become self-sufficient.

Bangladesh continues to get considerable food aid. In fact, the three-year average food aid received in 1992-93 was substantially more than the similar average in 1972-73 (Table 8.3). It is rather puzzling that despite a large increase in domestic production the volume of food aid has been increasing. However, if we take single year figures, the food aid in 1992-93 was only about half its previous year level and also the 1972-73 level. It seems that from now on Bangladesh may need only a small volume of food aid, except during emergencies. Bangladesh has become almost self-sufficient in meeting effective demand for rice, but wheat production is dropping because of the increasing area given to winter rice. I have already explained how the demand for wheat is increasing. Further, in the FFWP for the very poor in the rural areas, the wages are paid in wheat. The donor countries are keen to help Bangladesh in this very desirable program but they can only give food aid in wheat. It seems that since 1992-93 wheat aid also dropped by 50 percent and rice aid was only 20,000 tonnes.

180

Table 8.3
Food aid received by Bangladesh in 000 tonnes

Year	Rice	Wheat	Total Cereals
1971-72	199.2	410.9	610.1
1972-73	180.4	1029.0	1272.0
1973-74	83.5	570.9	660.3
1974-75	300.2	1775.8	2076.0
1975-76	323.4	851.0	1186.9
1976-77	90.4	904.4	994.8
1977-78	99.2	1164.6	1277.4
1978-79	153.0	1323.4	1496.6
1979-80	241.9	1235.8	1474.5
1980-81	88.1	645.4	736.9
1981-82	52.3	953.2	1005.5
1982-83	225.8	1026.5	1252.3
1983-84	150.2	1012.5	1162.7
1984-85	119.9	1380.1	1500.1
1985-86	23.6	1276.6	1300.3
1986-87	135.9	1451.0	1588.9
1987-88	165.5	1231.2	1396.6
1988-89	43.3	1276.7	1320.0
1989-90	41.1	1092.4	1133.5
1990-91	13.6	1342.7	1356.4
1991-92	23.2	1331.0	1354.1
1992-93	19.9	699.3	719.4

Source: Calculated by the author from BBS data

Bangladesh will continue to need food aid for some time to keep the FFWP going and for building reserve stocks. Because of its geographical location, Bangladesh will continue to be frequently affected by serious natural disasters and will need food aid. Land scarcity in Bangladesh is so acute that it cannot have large surplus production. It would be quite satisfying if it could only make ends meet.

Views about food aid are changing. Total food aid now amounts to less than 10 million tonnes per year, which is only a tiny fraction of the world trade in food. It seems that non-emergency food aid will decline in the future. In Bangladesh, there will be millions of people who will not be able to produce enough food for their own needs or to earn enough income to buy it. This aspect of the hunger problem is well tackled by the FFWP of the WFP. It is quite likely that Bangladesh will continue to get food aid for maintaining its FFWP.

The recent trend, on the other hand, is that emergency food aid will increase but other forms of aid will decline (Ingram 1988). On humanitarian grounds, Bangladesh will continue to get emergency food aid during serious natural disasters.

Entitlement protection and the state

As stated in the previous chapter, hunger is initiated by 'entitlement failure'. Therefore, the most important action for hunger alleviation should be entitlement protection. The governments play a major role in entitlement protection. In many developed and less developed countries governments operate several programs to protect the entitlements of vulnerable groups, e.g. through food subsidies, fixation of minimum wages, price control, and providing social security allowances to those who are out of work and those who are unable to work. Bangladesh has a long way to go in extending entitlement protection schemes to cover the majority of the poor and undernourished population, particularly in the rural areas. Bangladesh is surrounded by three regions, namely, China, Sri Lanka, and the Indian state of Kerala, where public action for hunger eradication has been very successful. Because Bangladesh depends heavily on American aid, adoption of Chinese model may not be quite acceptable to the donors. Nevertheless, public action for hunger eradication in Sri Lanka and Kerala are just as impressive, and provide a good model for Bangladesh to follow (Sudhir and Kanbur 1991). Both Kerala and Sri Lanka are widely quoted for their remarkable achievements in reducing hunger and mortality. In both cases, widespread literacy seems to have played an important role. In both places, primary education was given much more importance and funds and also much earlier than anywhere else in British India. Also, public distribution of subsidized food began in Sri Lanka as early as 1942. Now Sri Lanka has a variety of programs for improving the nutritional status of the poor. It distributes food to the poor through ration shops and food stamps at subsidized prices. In Kerala, the process started much later, but now it has an efficient system of distributing subsidized food through a network of ration shops, which cover much of the poor population in both urban and rural areas. A high level of literacy (both male and female), primary health care, and distribution of subsidized food have proved very successful in reducing mortality and hunger and collecting life expectancy well above the rest of South Asia (Bhattacharya, Chatterjee, and Pal 1988, Kumar 1987, Dreze and Sen 1989). In Bangladesh, the government operates several schemes for protecting food entitlements of the poor and not so poor[1]. It distributes subsidized food through a chain of ration shops, through FFWP, and also provides loans to small farmers and businesses. During emergencies, the government also distributes commodities and even money to the poor. But it cannot yet afford to have a social security program to look after those who cannot find work and those who are unable to work.

---

[1]The government and military employees.

In Bangladesh, there is a well established system for distributing subsidized food to the poor and not so poor. The system is called the Public Food Distribution System (PFDS). Since its introduction it has been expanded and modified several times. The PFDS has twelve channels for the distribution of subsidized food. It is, therefore, very clear that the government is strongly motivated to protect the entitlement of at least some selected groups. Of the twelve components of the PFDS, six are concerned with rationing but only two of the six rationing components operate on a regular basis and cover reasonably large sections of the population. These are Statutory Rationing (SR) and Modified Rationing (MR), each having a different objective. Most of the programs for the distribution of subsidized food are influenced by internal politics and the political and economic interests of the donor countries. The bulk of the food that is distributed as subsidized food is obtained as food aid. Therefore, the donor countries want to have a say in its distribution.

Food distribution through ration shops. The SR, in which subsidized food is distributed - sold at below market price - through ration shops, is the oldest entitlement protection program operating in Bangladesh. It was established during the Second World War in Bengal to cope with war-time scarcity. In its present form, it was designed to benefit selected urban population, i.e., public employees - civil and military - salaried workers of large scale industrial and commercial establishments, school teachers, high level businessmen, and professionals. Some low income wage earners such as artisans, rickshaw pullers, and domestic servants are also included in SR, but they account for only 6 percent of the card holders. No scrutiny of household incomes is done to decide legitimacy for SR. Clearly, the objective of SR has never been to protect the entitlement of the poor and to achieve some equity. It was designed to serve some political and administrative interests of the government. It looks at the food needs of those whose material well-being will ensure smooth running of the government machinery and national security. Chowdhury (1988)[2] found that the average income of the beneficiaries of SR was significantly above average. A good majority of them have well paid and secure government jobs, and are not very protective of their SR entitlements. For example, an adult unit on as SR card carries an entitlement of 1.5 kg of wheat and 0.5 kg of rice per day; the entitlement of a minor unit is half that much. But very often, when minors turn adults in SR households, the card holders do not promptly get the quota for minors upgraded. Some card holders do not get the quota upgraded at all (Chowdhury 1988). Also, many card holders use less than 60 percent of their full ration entitlement, but the allotment of rice collected is much greater than that of wheat.

The main reason why the urban elites are chosen to benefit from SR is that they are politically powerful. They not only have considerable voting power in the cities, but also the ability to influence voting behaviour in rural areas. Many urban elites

---

[2]The section on rationing is based rather heavily on Chowdhury 1986 and 1988.

own agricultural land in villages, and they have it cultivated by tenant farmers. They are also the intelligentsia of the nation, and therefore have the ability to use media and organize demonstrations against the government, if dissatisfied with their living conditions. The government policy, therefore, is to win their support by keeping them happy and satisfied.

The SR covers six cities, namely Dhaka, Chittagong, Narayanganj, Khulna, Rajshahi, and Rangamati. Rangamati was the last to join the group in 1975. The chosen households in these cities were issued cards up until 1975. Since then new cards have not been issued, except to the households of the government employees who were transferred to any of the six cities from other parts of the country. The present holders of SR ration cards have long residential status in cities. This implies that many rural households who moved into cities have not been included in SR. A large majority of those who move into cities from villages are landless labourers or small farmers and definitely deserve some support, but unfortunately they are excluded. The largest concentration of SR card holders is in Dhaka and Khulna cities, which account for about 70 percent of all SR members.

Over time, several changes have occurred in the SR of Bangladesh. First of all, its importance seems to be declining. The share of SR in the total quantity of food distributed through PFDS dropped from 23.4 in 1973-74 to 13.0 percent in 1983-84. The quantity of rice and wheat distributed in 1984-85 through SR had dropped to almost half its level in 1973-74, but during the same period the quantity of the two cereals distributed through PFDS increased by 25 percent. Hence, the share of food distribution through SR in PFDS appears to be declining. Another notable change in SR is the drop in the price of rice and an increase in the price of wheat (Table 8.4). In the early 1970s, SR was very attractive because the difference between ration price and market price was much greater than it was in the mid 1980s. The decline in the price difference has affected the proportion of the allotment collected by SR households. By paying more, the SAR households can pick and choose from a larger variety of rice and other food items. Those in the higher income groups do not seem to mind paying more for better quality.

For several reasons, SR in Bangladesh is subject to misuse. It is estimated that up to 40 percent of the foodgrains supplied for distribution represent potential leakage. The leakage occurs at two points, i.e., at the ration shops and at the households. Because ration shop prices are significantly lower than market prices, even after dropping over time, there is a great temptation for the ration shop-keepers to sell whatever quantity they can manage in the open market. They make very attractive profit — about 70 percent more than what the government allows them to make on the issue price (Chowdhury 1988). The leakage is made easier for shopkeepers because considerable stock is not collected by card holders. The leakage at the household level occurs because the allotment quota is very high. In SR households 30 to 40 percent of the food expenditure is on meat and fish, and therefore the quantity of foodgrains consumed is relatively small. By comparing the

Table 8.4
Issue prices of selected rationed commodities in the month of June in Takas per kilogram from 1974 to 1986

Year	Rice	Wheat	Rape seed oil	Ghee
1974	1.61	1.34	8.57	10.20
1975	1.61	1.34	8.57	10.20
1977	2.41	1.87	10.72	12.86
1978	2.68	2.14	13.93	15.00
1979	3.21	2.41	13.93	17.15
1981	4.15	3.11	13.93	17.15
1982	5.22	3.59	13.93	25.72
1983	11.34	7.66	27.42	51.38
1984	15.25	8.17	39.37	70.87
1986	15.25	10.14	39.37	70.87

Source: Compiled by the author from BBS data

foodgrains collected by SR households and the quantity consumed, it was noted that 18 percent of the foodgrains collected could not be accounted for. It is rather puzzling to note that households do not collect all their quota and yet presumably sell part of what they collect at a handsome profit in the open market. Thus, a few explanatory statements made above for leakage are inadequate. The real reason may be quite complex and at present not known. One thing appears quite clear, that the distribution of much of the food through SR mostly goes to those who are not undernourished.

Despite its various weaknesses, SR has made a significant improvement in the nutritional intake of those ration card holders who are in lower income groups. Several categories of low income government employees such as cleaners, watchmen, junior clerks, transport workers, and labourers in large scale establishments, who are also entitled to SR, have benefited significantly. Further, due perhaps to better utilization of SR benefits by those in lower income groups, there has been some improvement in income distribution.

Modified Rationing (MR) was added to the PFDS in 1949. It was realized quite early in the history of rationing that SR was not doing anything to reduce hunger in the rural areas where hunger was most concentrated. Now MR distributes subsidized foodgrains to low income households in rural areas and urban municipalities not covered by SR. Households are classified into four categories according to *chowkidari* tax[3] which they pay. The bottom two categories are entitled to get all

[3] The tax paid by rural households for keeping a watch on their property at night. Each village employs a night watchman.

the benefits of the MR, but those in the upper two categories are entitled to only some non-cereal items. The ration prices and quotas per card are the same in MR as in SR. But the government allocates more foodgrains to MR when open market prices are high (Montgomery 1985). In reality, actual distribution is not based on maximum allowable quotas. Therefore, members of MR continually keep trying to move into other priority groups.

Since Bangladesh became independent, the structure of PFDS has again undergone several changes. For example, the status of MR and SR dropped considerably between 1973-74 and 1983-84. The decline for MR and SR was 58 and 44 percent respectively. It seems that FFWP has become the more popular and accepted method of hunger alleviation or entitlement protection. During the period between 1973-74 and 1983-84, distribution of subsidized food increased by 950 percent. The MR has several weaknesses because of which the full benefits of the program do not reach the target groups. For example, the district priority lists (DPL) are not revised frequently enough. Therefore, new eligible households are deprived of the benefits for long durations, sometimes for more than five years (Chowdhury 1988). Therefore, those who are in the MR may deserve the benefit of the scheme, but a large number of those who should be entitled to the benefit are left out. The administrative inefficiency unnecessarily adds to the misery of the undernourished. There is also some doubt concerning the fairness in the selection of households for MR benefits. Further, the method used for the selection of households to benefit from MR is so stringent that even if all households that satisfied the criteria were included, only 11.5 percent of the rural poor would benefit. Although it was designed to protect the food entitlement of the rural poor, in practice it benefits only a very small percentage of the rural poor. Also, in the actual distribution of foodgrains, the rural poor are again discriminated against relative to the households in municipalities. The urban households, on an average for Bangladesh, get almost four times more per card. The leakage in MR is just as bad as in SR.

Some simple modifications to the scheme, suggested below, would make it more effective in alleviating hunger, without doing any damage to the political objectives of the scheme. First, the criteria set for the selection of households should be made more generous so that more low income households become qualified for holding a ration card. This is not likely to increase the burden on the government for increasing the supply of subsidized food to the ration shops, because existing supplies are not fully collected by the card holders. Apparently, the existing supplies should be adequate for a considerably larger population of beneficiaries, if fully collected. Further, surveys conducted by Chowdhury (1988) also reveal that the existing quotas are too high and can be reduced without harming the card holders. Hence, the second modification should be to set new quotas at more realistic levels. A careful sample survey of card holders may be required to determine their actual needs of foodgrains. The results of the survey will help to fix new and more realistic quota limits. However, some adjustments to the survey results may be necessary to rectify the exaggerated claims of some respondents. The new quotas may still allow

186

card holders to collect the same quantity as they are collecting at present, but they may have to collect nearly their full entitlements. These two modifications will considerably clean up the system by stopping leakage. As card holders begin to collect their full quotas, there will be less left with the shopkeepers for leakage. Also, by making quotas commensurate with the needs of card holders, there will be less left with the households to sell in the open market.

Food for work program   The government in Bangladesh, like most other governments in Third World countries, also protects entitlements by providing employment to a large number of people in the public sector. Often, a high proportion of those who work in the public sector may be regarded as redundant, because their sacking would have no impact on productivity (Sobhan 1990). But the government keeps them employed for political reasons. It keeps unemployment down and lessens social tension. But most of the government activities are concentrated in the cities, and therefore do not help create employment for the rural poor. As hunger and poverty are most concentrated in rural areas, the government introduced the Rural Works Program (RWP) to provide some employment to the rural poor for protecting their food entitlement. The rural poor are given foodgrains instead of money wages for work on selected rural projects. The main objectives of the program are to alleviate hunger and at the same time build rural infrastructure such as roads, embankments, irrigation and drainage canals etc.

The rural RWPs have been operating in Bangladesh for quite some time. They have been chopped and changed so frequently that we now have six different types of RWPs operating in the country.[4] Although each one of the six programs is concerned with reduction of hunger and poverty in rural areas, and therefore directly or indirectly with entitlement protection, the most important among them in magnitude and geographical coverage is the Food For Work Program (FFWP). It began after the 1974 famine. During the famine the government opened about 6,000 gruel kitchens to feed the affected population. After the famine, the government felt the need for providing relief from hunger on a more regular basis through FFWP. The FFWP depends almost entirely on overseas donations of wheat, which are coordinated by WFP and CARE. The main donors are the USA, Canada, the UK, and Australia. The projects undertaken for construction are nominated by various government and local area organizations. In the mid 1980s, they were dominated by the BWDB and the Ministry of Relief and Rehabilitation (MRR). In 1983-84, out of roughly 2,000 projects about 90 percent were reconstructions of existing facilities that had deteriorated over time, and only 10 percent were new projects (Asaduzzaman and Huddleston 1983). Road construction, river embankments, and re-excavation of irrigation and drainage canals dominated the list of projects under FFWP contracts.

An outstanding feature of FFWP is a high degree of local participation in the

---

[4] These are : the original RWP, the Special Public Works Program, the Food For Work Program, the Intensive Rural Works Program, the Early Implementation Program, and the Zila Road Maintenance Program.

selection of projects. Local participation in planning and development is advantageous if it truly represents the local needs of the majority. But sometimes it may end in the selection of projects not properly conceived and may represent the interests of a few big landowners, who are locally influential and politically powerful.

The wages are paid in wheat for a prescribed piece of work. The prescribed rate of wage payment is 43 seers of wheat for 1,000 cubic feet of earthwork. There are other standards employed for payment of wages where the work cannot be measured according to the volume of earthwork. A notable feature of wage payment is that women get a higher wage for the same amount of work (Asaduzzman and Huddleston 1983).

The regional distribution of projects under FFWP is quite uneven. There is a marked concentration of projects in Rangpur, Barisal, Faridpur, and Sylhet districts, and a lack of concentration in Pabna, Bogra, and Jamalpur. There appears to be a greater concentration of FFWP projects in the more flood-prone districts, where there is greater need for reconstruction and maintenance of canals, embankments, roads, and small bridges.

A management survey conducted jointly by the Bangladesh Institute of Development Studies and the International Food Policy Research Institute in 1982 revealed some mismanagement of wheat stocks donated by various countries. It was estimated that at least 15 percent of the wheat stocks disappear from the Local Storage Depots (LSD). The disappearance is made up under payment to actual workers. Also, estimates of work involved in projects are exaggerated in order to claim more wheat than is actually required. Some wheat, it was reported, was also sold to cover unjustified payments to officials who approve the initial submissions for project costs and who inspect project sites.

Hossain and Asaduzzman (1983) estimated the benefits of several projects completed under FFWP and RWP, and found that the projects were yielding many benefits to the rural communities. They found that even the construction of *Kuthca* (unsealed) roads was beneficial. The volume to goods transported by vehicular transport increased and costs dropped.

The FFWP requires large resources and without external help it would be impossible to sustain it in Bangladesh. It is largely funded by WFP, US aid, Canadian aid, Australian aid, domestic surplus, and occasionally by some other countries. In the FFWP, food is given directly to the needy for work. It bypasses the middlemen. The direct payment of foodgrains instead of cash to the rural poor keeps the demand low and therefore prices down. Hence, the program helps in yet another way to protect the entitlement of the poor. However, it is criticised for its negative effect on foodgrain prices, which dampens the incentive to increase domestic production. Some have also argued that the FFWP provides only short-term employment and is therefore unlikely to make any permanent improvement in the living standards of the poor. Although the projects chosen in the FFWP mostly help landowners because they are focused on agricultural development, they do have a significant impact on hunger alleviation. This is because agricultural development in the long run will have some spin-offs that will benefit the poor, for example, more employment not only in agriculture but in several other related activities.

The government also plays an important role in entitlement protection through procurement of foodgrains at guarantied prices from producers and releasing them when there is some scarcity. In this way the government holds some control over food prices and protects the food entitlements of the poor. Food supply by its very nature suffers from a great deal of uncertainty, because it depends on natural and economic variables which are not fixed. This holds for both developed and developing countries. Even a country like Australia, which is a major wheat exporting country, had to import wheat in 1994, due to widespread crop failure. Therefore, food storage is essential to avoid hunger and starvation. Even hunters and gatherers with their rudimentary technology had developed some methods for food storage (Garine and Harrison 1988). Over the years in Bangladesh, the government has built an extensive system of food storage. There are two types of government food storage godowns and silos, i.e., Local Supply Depots and Central Supply Depots. In 1991, the total capacity of the two was around 1.7 million tonnes. The storage capacity is well distributed throughout the country, but there is some noticeable concentration in the more urban districts. As the urban population entirely depends on rural food production and imports, there is greater need for reserve stocks in the urban districts in times of scarcity. Hence, the largest storage capacity is found in the three most urbanized districts, namely, Dhaka, Chittagong, and Khulna. Also, more than average storage capacity is provided in the surplus western districts, probably to reduce transport costs. The most urgent need for providing food to the very poor comes when some part of the country is hit by a serious natural disaster, for example when standing crops, ready for harvesting, are suddenly wiped off by a cyclone or flash floods. Such events immediately lead to a sudden rise in food prices, putting food beyond the reach of many who in normal times could manage to buy barely enough for their needs. Hence, the number of those who need food relief suddenly increases several fold after disasters. Therefore, direct delivery of food in large quantities is required to feed those who have lost their exchange entitlement. Of course, the international community is always very prompt in giving food aid in such emergencies, but it takes time, sometime weeks, before food begins to arrive from overseas. Immediate feeding of the destitute population is always the responsibility of the domestic organizations and depends on domestic resources.

Because food supply depends to a very large extent on natural factors over which people have no control, it is subject to fluctuations everywhere. But in some regions such as Bangladesh, the food supply fluctuates much more. The storage of reserve stocks of foodgrains is essential and a very effective method of providing immediate food relief. Therefore, Bangladesh confronts an enormous problem of producing enough food not only for a population which is increasing in size and affluency but also for building reserve stocks. Considering the severe limitations of land, which is decreasing in size due to erosion particularly of river banks, to achieve that level of food self-sufficiency from the agricultural sector alone will be difficult indeed. It will be essential to develop a strong export-oriented manufacturing sector. From the export of manufactures it will then be possible to import additional food, like most countries of Europe and several in Asia do. There is considerable potential for several manufacturing industries in Bangladesh, such as jute products, textiles, food processing, and other labour intensive industries. Some of these are already operating successfully in Bangladesh.

Entitlement protection and the non-government organizations

Although it is abundantly clear that the government has a genuine interest in the reduction of hunger and poverty, its efforts have not been very effective for several reasons. The government sector is overstaffed for political reasons. As stated earlier, a considerable reduction in the workforce may not make much difference in productivity. The employees, although under-paid, are happy because they have employment and access to several benefits other than their salaries. The government is satisfied with the arrangement because it reduces the chances of political unrest. Hence, the level of efficiency in several projects is low. Further, there are also serious resource constraints that prevent the government from launching projects to meet the basic social needs of all. The annual budget of Bangladesh shows how badly the government depends on foreign aid. Therefore, some observers believe that high levels of hunger and poverty may remain in Bangladesh for several decades. The government, therefore, seeks the help of Non-Government Organizations (NGOs) in hunger and poverty eradication programs. The help of NGOs is desperately needed in several areas but most importantly for further expansion of health, education, and nutrition facilities and in making villages more accessible for aid to reach them. However, there are groups within Bangladesh, particularly those inclined towards the political left, who criticise the work of NGOs on the grounds that they are making Bangladesh more dependent on foreign countries and diverting the government's attention from its main responsibility of providing the basic needs of all people. Nevertheless, the NGOs are operating in Bangladesh and doing commendable work. The number of indigenous NGOs now operating in Bangladesh is over 200, and an additional 60 are international (Lovell 1992). Some of the indigenous NGOs are very small and only cover small areas. Similarly, some of the international NGOs are small and inconsistent, and some have ceased operations.

The Bangladesh Rural Advancement Committee (BRAC) is the largest indigenous NGO that is involved in hunger and poverty eradication in Bangladesh. It was founded by Fagel H. Abed, who is now the executive director of the organization. It began in 1970 as a small emergency food aid venture. BRAC is largely funded by international NGOs. It depends on foreign donors to the tune of 85 percent of its annual budget. The track record of BRAC is very impressive. One reason for BRAC's outstanding success is that it takes more risk in making investments in various programs. They accept that some programs may fail. Nevertheless, the success rate is very high. It covers a large area and population, and has won the confidence of external NGOs, who provide financial support to it, such as the Netherlands Organization of International Development Corporation (NOVIB), the Swiss Development Corporation (SDC), the Swiss International Development Agency (SIDA), EZE of Germany, and several others mentioned in Table 8.5. Oxfam (British, Canada, and US), UNICEF, SDC, EZE, Ford Foundation, Bread for the World, and NOVIB are some of the more consistent donors to BRAC. There are several smaller contributors who for some reason have stopped donations in the 1980s. The work of NGOs has been so good that several foreign aid donors to Bangladesh have started giving aid directly to NGOs.

Table 8.5
Ten leading NGOs supporting BRAC's hunger and poverty alleviation programs

Name	Total paid between 1972 and 1990 (Million US $)
Netherlands Organization for International Development Corporation (NOVIB)	17.20
Swiss Development Corporation (SDC)	5.52
Swiss International Development Agency (SIDA)	5.02
Evangelische Zentralstelle Fur Entwicklumgshilfe (EZE Germany)	4.99
UNICEF	4.99
British Overseas Development Agency (ODA)	4.23
Danish International Development Agency (DNIDA)	2.62
Norwegian Aid Agency (NORAD)	1.86
Swedish Free Church Aid (SFCA)	1.54
Ford Foundation	1.21

Source: Adapted from Lovell 1992

BRAC and some other NGOs who work independently concentrate particularly on the rural poor who are not benefited by the government poverty alleviation programs. They focus on the landless poor population, particularly on rural women who are destitute, old, deserted, and handicapped. Their main objective is to reach the grass roots. BRAC particularly believes that even illiterate and very poor asset-less individuals can rise and contribute to solving their own problems, sometimes without any financial support, if given the opportunities, encouragement, and proper guidance. BRAC also stresses the importance of women in poverty and hunger alleviation, because they are as yet not corrupt and are very responsible borrowers.

BRAC operates at the village level. They have a village office for 40 to 50 villages, and each office covers about 100 village organizations. In each selected village 2 or 3 village organizations are created to organize the poor into sub-groups consisting of households. In each village office, there are three Program Organizers (POs). Often the POs are fresh university graduates from the local areas, who are unemployed and therefore willing to work on low wages. Before going to the field, the POs are given short training in BRAC's own establishments. BRAC spends considerable funds on the training and upgrading of its own staff. Each PO is assisted by three *gram sevaks* (GS)[5]. The GS are young villagers who are very familiar with the village problems. All staff of a village office live together, eat together, and conduct regular meetings to discuss the problems of the selected villages. Hence, BRAC's strategy is to involve the beneficiaries in the actual work and also decision making.

BRAC operates many 'non-formal' primary education centres in selected villages. Besides adult literacy, the education centres run by BRAC focus on 'functional education', which emphasises the village problems and their solutions. Another objective of functional education is to make the rural poor informed about their environment and their political and legal rights. The BRAC education centres teach villagers what they should do if they are illegally harassed by the police, other government officers, and other villagers. These centres also provide a rare opportunity for the rural poor to sit down and discuss their own problems and how to solve them. Thus, the poor are able to think of mobilizing their own power and resources and stand together against violation of their social and political rights.

The economic programs are focused on income generation for the vulnerable groups. They include household poultry programs, rural credit programs, and credit for very small businesses. Household poultry programs are particularly successful. They requires little training and costs, and also marketing of the output is easy. Only a few chicks are given to a household to raise them for laying eggs. A small cage is provided. Some women in the village are trained for vaccinating the chicks against disease. For a household poultry program, women are given small loans for feed, for buying HYV chicks, and for the cage. Once the venture begins yielding income the women's groups or households commence repayments of loans.

BRAC also gives wheat rations to some women who are very poor, deserted, and have children to support. Such women get a ration of 31.25 kg of wheat for a two-year period. If they are physically reasonably fit, they are put on some income-generating program and become self-supporting within the two-year period. BRAC also runs an outreach program to provide guidance and advice to some rural poor. It is based on the belief that some poor individuals can be uplifted if only they can be motivated to better utilize their own resources.

BRAC is the most effective indigenous NGO operating in Bangladesh, but its external dependence has become very high (85 percent). BRAC is quite conscious about its high foreign dependency and is making efforts to reduce it. It is now building up commercial enterprises which will generate some income for the organization. The Rural Credit Project, which has now become the BRAC Bank, is fully self-supporting through interest income. BRAC has been successful in encouraging poor villagers to save and invest in income generating programs. By mid 1990, the rural poor had saved more than Tk. 100 million for investment in their own income-generating programs (Lovell 1992).

There are several other NGOs operating in Bangladesh. The major objective of all NGOs is the same, i.e., alleviation of hunger and poverty, particularly in the rural areas. Most of the NGOs operating in Bangladesh are non-religious charitable organizations, but some are supported largely by religious bodies. Here we will take a case study of one such NGO, called CARITAS, which is operating very successfully in Bangladesh. CARITAS was initiated by the Catholic Bishops Conference, held in Bangladesh in 1973. CARITAS is now funded by a large number of donors largely from European Catholic and non-Catholic organizations. The main goal initially was to increase food production. However, the realization that increasing food production is dependent upon several other developments has broadened the scope of the CARITAS program considerably. The main objective now appears to be the fulfilment of the basic needs of the people and uplifting their social and nutritional status. But the initial objective of increasing food production and feeding the vulnerable groups is still carried out as enthusiastically as before. CARITAS is directly involved in increasing food production. It runs land reclamation, irrigation, agricultural education, fish culture, and vegetable and fruit farming programs. Fish culture is an ideal means of increasing food supply in Bangladesh, particularly for small farmers whose lands are adversely affected by low and medium level floods. A portion of the field or even the entire field can be converted into a fish pond. The earth taken out from the diggings is spread around the edges of the pond to make high embankments, to protect the pond from low and medium level floods. The field begins to produce fish instead of crops. The income derived from fish is much more than from any food crop. On an average a fish farming yields Tk 36,000 per acre. The embankments are used for fruit and vegetable farming and give additional income. CARITAS has established fish farming projects in 24 *upzilas*. All have proved very successful. In 1995, there were more than 700 fish ponds spread over 207 acres.

During emergencies, CARITAS distributes food items such as rice, pulses, potatoes, sugar, salt, etc. free to victims. In addition to food a variety of essential non-food items are also distributed free (Table 8.6). After a natural disaster, the majority of the poor, who do not have proper shelter, are completely dislocated. Often they lose everything. Therefore, they need not only food but clothing, cooking utensils, and something to protect their belongings that they have been able to save and what they get from relief agencies.

CARITAS is also involved in direct feeding and food distribution, during normal times, to the very poor who are incapable of working, and to those who are old, sick, invalid or handicapped in some other way. The feeding centres are run with the help of WFP. A group of undernourished children are chosen from a village and are put on a special feeding program. After sufficient improvement in their nutritional status, the group is taken out of the program and is replaced by a new group. In the nutrition program, the parents of children who are taken into special feeding

193

programs are given instructions in nutrition. They are informed about the nutritional values of easily available foods, and how to prepare nutritional meals at low cost.

Table 8.6
List of selected essential articles distributed free to 1991 cyclone victims by CARITAS

Items	Quantity	
Food articles		
Rice	123, 951	Kg.
Pulses	32, 240	"
Salt	5, 773	"
Potatoes	59, 739	"
Sugar	1, 700	"
Milk powder	400	Bags
Clothing articles		
Sarees	15, 484	Nos.
Lungi (Cloth rapped around lower portion of the body by men)	16, 320	"
Gamcha (Thin towel)	14, 520	"
Second hand clothes	6	Bales
Household articles		
Plastic bowls	3, 000	Nos
Cooking utensils	101, 740	"
Containers	5,108	"
Kerosene	9, 392	Litres
Blankets and quilts	133	Bales
Plastic sheets	8, 810	Pieces
Bandages	30	Drums
Water purifying tablets	2.5	Million

Source: CARITAS, News Letter, March 1992

CARITAS, like other NGOs and the government, realizes that increasing the food purchasing power of the poor is essential for hunger eradication. It runs a Rural Works Program (RWP). The main objective of the program is to create income-

194

earning opportunities for the landless poor households, and to expand rural infrastructure through self-help projects. The projects chosen are those that are considered most important by the majority of the local population. The beneficiaries pay 20 percent of the cost of a selected project. Those who get work in a project are paid wages in cash. In this respect, the CARITAS work program is distinctly different from FFWP run by the government. CARITAS believes that poor people need money, not wheat, for buying food of their choice. Many households in FFWP have to sell all or at least part of the wheat they get as wages, in order to buy some food and other essentials, and lose the value of their wages in the process. The projects undertaken by the RPW are construction of roads, culverts, small bridges, irrigation canals, embankments, re-excavation of silted ponds, pit latrines etc.

CARITAS believes that without uplifting the social status of the rural poor, particularly women, there can be no permanent solution to hunger. Therefore, several of its programs are focused on improving the social and economic status of the landless rural poor. First of all, it is essential to provide permanent accommodation for the rural poor. Without a permanent place to live, a household cannot be free from hunger. Therefore, CARITAS is actively involved in the construction of low cost houses and emergency community shelters. The low cost houses are built of bamboo mat walls and C.I. sheet roofs. They are made on sufficiently raised ground to avoid damage during low and medium level floods. They consist of one or two rooms, cooking space, and a pit latrine. A large number of low cost houses have been built in 7 districts, where CARITAS operates or has regional centres. In addition to low cost housing, CARITAS has also constructed 142 reinforced concrete community cyclone shelters. They are located in the high risk coastal zones from Chittagong to Khulna.

The third area of serious concern is rural literacy, education, vocational training, and health. CARITAS runs literacy centres for adults, and feeder schools for pre-school children to develop school-going habits among destitute and slum children. Feeder schools also make mothers free to go to literacy classes or to some income-earning training course. Children are also provided with medical and preventive health care services. The vocational training schools for men and women offer training in accountancy, electrical trades, T.V. and radio repairs, plumbing, carpentry etc. All literacy, education, and training programs are specially focused on women, because they are grossly discriminated against in Bangladesh. Discrimination starts from birth. Male children are better fed and cared for than female children. The female children are, therefore, more undernourished. The level of literacy is also lower among women.

One important element of the CARITAS development philosophy is that they make the beneficiaries pay part of the cost of a project. For example, in fish farming, beneficiaries pay 7 percent of the cost of a fish pond. In other rural projects under RWP, they pay 20 percent of the cost. This makes the beneficiaries more interested in the projects undertaken.

The indigenous and overseas NGOs are certainly helping the government in its poverty alleviation programs. In some areas the contribution of NGOs is more than that of the government. For example, in Manpura Island, the number of schools and cyclone shelters built and run by the NGOs stands higher than that by the government.

While discussing the role of government and non-government organizations in hunger reduction and entitlement protection, the work of the Grameen Bank should not be overlooked. The Grameen Bank is a quasi-government organization. The contribution of the Grameen Bank in entitlement protection through promotion of small scale self-employment for the rural poor is now widely recognized. The bank has been amazingly successful in enabling landless rural poor to become self-employed in income-generating non-agricultural activities. The landless poor have the capacity to become gainfully employed in trading, shopkeeping, and manufacturing of handicrafts, if given some starting capital. But they cannot get credit from the scheduled banks because they have no assets, and therefore they are not regarded as credit worthy. The Grameen Bank took an unusual step in introducing a scheme to give small credit to asset-less households for starting small scale income-earning activities.

The large majority of the beneficiaries are landless and were unemployed before becoming self-employed with the help of the Grameen Bank. The target population for giving credit is any unemployed member of a household that owns less than half an acre of land. The bank covered only about 15 percent of the target population in only 6 percent of the villages (Osmani 1989). In 1992, it had 1.4 million landless members of which 1.3 million were women. It is still a small organization and therefore has not yet confronted the problems faced by large organizations.

The Grameen Bank is especially committed to raising the status of women. In 1986, 74 percent of the loanees were women (Hossain 1988). In 1992, the percentage of women increased to 93. Women have been found to be more responsible borrowers. A large number of women, with the credit received from the bank, are now running their own small businesses, and contributing significantly to the household incomes. Within the households of the beneficiaries, female participation in the labour force increased from 5 to 25 percent within a short period. Women also stand out prominently as bank employees.

The Grameen Bank's philosophy is that the poor are capable of helping themselves. They are clever and have a clear idea of the income-earning opportunities in their local regions. They also know which of the opportunities are within their reach, considering the limitations of their own education, training, experience, and physical abilities. But they need some financial assistance to start an income-earning venture that is otherwise within their capacity. Therefore the bank strongly depends on the initiative of the beneficiaries in choosing a project. An individual first makes a proposal to the bank for starting a small income earning venture. If the applicant is not literate, he or she simply has to describe the project to a bank officer. There are no forms to be filled. After examining the proposal very carefully, the bank officers visit the household and ascertain the capabilities of the applicant for the proposed project. If satisfied, the bank asks the applicant to form a group of five loanees, although the loan is given to an individual who alone is responsible for repayments. But a default by any one in the group disqualifies all members for any further loans from the bank. Therefore, all members of a group keep a close watch on each other for regular and timely repayments of instalments. There are also weekly meetings conducted to discuss progress of the projects and repayments in each village. If a defaulter's name is mentioned in a meeting, it is a matter of insult. So, the bank's strategy is to put group and social pressure on the loanees for regular repayments of weekly instalments. The bank allows sufficient time for the project to get going before asking for repayments. Repayments begin when the venture begins yielding some income.

The Grameen bank is not a charitable organization. It firmly believes that giving handouts to the poor is not going to help them on a permanent basis. The bank operates on purely banking principles. It charges relatively high interest of 18 percent on all loans, because it gives loans without any security and takes higher risks of bad debts. But the recovery rate is above 80 percent which is quite high.

A survey conducted in 1985 indicated that the average income of the beneficiary households was 43 percent higher than the non-beneficiary households of the target population, but initially it was not so (Hossain 1988). The beneficiaries were certainly enjoying a higher standard of living than their non-beneficiary counterparts in the target population. The survey also revealed that in most of the non-agricultural trading and some manufacturing activities the return to family labour was higher than agricultural wage rates in the local region. But in cattle and poultry raising and some handicraft manufacturing the returns to family labour were lower than agricultural wages. However, these latter activities are predominantly carried out by women, who do not find much employment in agriculture. Thus, even though they may be getting less for their labour than in agriculture, their income is a net addition to family income.

The Grameen Bank is certainly collecting the food entitlements of the participating households and enabling them to rise above the poverty level. Many participating households are now enjoying a higher standard of living than before.

Beyond hunger

To solve the hunger problem on a permanent basis, a lot more than simply providing enough food for the existing population will have to be done. A new social and economic environment will have to be created, which will ensure enough food for all. Such an environment will have to have different set of priorities. For example, policies stressing participatory economic growth are necessary, i.e., growth policies in which a good majority of population will be able to participate (Dreze and Sen 1989). Such policies are likely to be based on labour intensive methods of production in the initial stages of growth so that the benefits of growth are more widely distributed. Policies to create such an environment will have to be introduced simultaneously with policies designed to increase food production and to increase or at least protect the food exchange entitlement of the vulnerable groups. The policies will have to concentrate on raising the quality of human resources in order to improve the capabilities of the labour force for assuming responsibilities in vocations demanding greater skills than agriculture and manual labouring. This implies the creation of a healthy and more educated community. Health and education both have a profound influence on the standard of living of a community and therefore on their nutritional status.

Education will have both short-term and long-term effects on the nutritional intake of people. The immediate effects will be those related to better knowledge of nutrition. For example, an educated housewife will have greater success in providing a low cost but more nutritious diet to the household than an uneducated one. Also, she will determine expenditure priorities in such a way that the basic needs will be fulfilled first. The members of the household will be better fed and clothed within a given income. She will, therefore, be able to stretch the given income further by judicious planning of the family budget.

Basic education will have several other indirect effects on the family income and therefore on the nutritional status of the family members. It will enable a household to avoid to a considerable extent several common diseases that result from lack of personal hygiene and sanitation. This will augment household income by reducing time away from work due to illness.

Basic education will help the poor in augmenting their incomes in several other ways. It will help small farmers in understanding and participating in new cultivation techniques, in keeping proper records of finances and input and output relationships, in making right tenurial contracts when leasing in land, and in avoiding unnecessary harassment for money lenders and landlords. It will also increase their access to available credit facilities, because they will be more informed about their rights and able to make proper applications for loans. The expansion of basic education will lay the foundation for a greater flow of young people into higher and technical education. It will expose the hidden talent of the community, raise the level of skills of the workforce, and prepare it for vocations that yield higher incomes.

Finally, an educated community will be more exposed to the economic and political system of the country. It will have a greater capacity for mobilization of forces to make their voices heard. The politicians, therefore, will not be able to easily by-pass them, as they often do with the groups who are of no political significance.

The general health of the community is just as important as education in hunger alleviation. There is a circular relationship between health and undernutrition. Prolonged undernutrition exerts a negative influence on mental and physical development. It impairs working and learning capacities of individuals, and lowers their income earning capacities. Therefore, undernourished people are more commonly found among low income occupations, the unemployed, and old people unable to work. Low incomes reduce access to food and keep people physically weak and intellectually underdeveloped (Lampty and Sai 1985). Hence, undernourished people remain permanently in poor health and in low income activities. Many experts believe that undernutrition (particularly protein-calorie malnutrition) in the first five years of life causes irreparable damage to mental development. Also physical weakness caused by undernutrition leads to a low resistance to disease. Several diseases of the digestive system such as gastroenteritis, diarrhoea, and chronic dysentery reduce food-holding capacity and make people even more undernourished. The little food that they can afford does not do much good to the body. The undernourished and physically weak people are more exposed to infections due to poor resistance. There is evidence that in times of epidemics large numbers of low income undernourished people die, reducing labour supply immensely. Such a drastic drop in labour supply often completely wipes out food supply and cause local famines (Lampty and Sai 1985). Therefore, improvement and considerable expansion of health services must be an integral part of a policy to alleviate hunger. In Bangladesh, although there has been considerable improvement in health services, the rural areas continue to suffer from inadequate health services. The percentage of GDP spent on health facilities has consistently increased throughout the 1980s and early 1990s. Nevertheless the percentage is very low, being less than 2 percent.

Summary

Increasing domestic food supply and at the same time increasing the food purchasing power of the poor are the two most important prerequisites for hunger alleviation. The government of Bangladesh is strongly committed to achieving self-sufficiency in food supply and reduction of hunger. Hence, it has played a major role in promoting infrastructure required for agricultural development. The infrastructure for development was gravely lacking in Bangladesh due to lack of genuine interest in the country during the British and the Pakistani regimes. The development of minor and major irrigation and the distribution of modern agricultural inputs at subsidised prices for the promotion of HYRVs played the most important role in increasing domestic food supply.

The government policy for the reduction of hunger and poverty is often criticised for not doing enough in the area of land reform to reduce inequality in the distribution of land resources, which would have made hunger reduction more effective. But this is debatable. Some scholars think that any program to redistribute land would have created more problems without much change in hunger and poverty. This may be true, but something certainly could have been done to protect the interests of the tenant farmers and to stop fragmentation of holdings. The government policy in Bangladesh definitely failed in improving agricultural structure and tenancy laws. The schemes for the protection of food exchange entitlement, such as public food distribution through ration shops and FFWP, are inadequate and do not cover the majority of the undernourished population. The subsidised rationing scheme suffers from urban bias for political reasons and mainly benefits those who really do not need it and, in fact, do not utilize their full entitlement. Only 6 percent of the ration-card-holders in the urban areas are low income earners, and the poor in the rural areas are badly neglected. The FFWP, launched in rural areas recently, is now helping to improve the rural infrastructure and also helping the rural poor. However, the effectiveness of both the schemes — FFWP and rationing — is marred by urban bias, political motives, and administrative corruption.

The government's ability to expand further the food exchange entitlement protection schemes is limited mainly due to lack of resources and a low level of efficiency in the government-run projects. The government has, therefore, welcomed the help of NGOs in hunger and poverty eradication programs. The NGOs are making an important contribution to improvements in health, education, and the nutritional status of the rural poor. BRAC is the largest indigenous NGO. It has now gained international recognition in lifting the living standards of the poorest of the rural poor by giving them small loans for starting small income-generating ventures. The international NGOs are just as important.

9 Summary and conclusion

The future of Bangladesh continues to appear very gloomy to those who are not aware of the latest developments in food production and consumption in Bangladesh. They continue to think of Bangladesh as an over-populated and resource poor country, where all efforts to alleviate hunger and poverty are foiled by frequent natural disasters. This image was formed after the 1974 famine in which more than 100,000 people died, and since then frequent cries for food aid after every natural disaster have dominated people's mind. The reality is far different. In the shadow of a vulnerable environment a new nation is emerging, where in the near future people will live in dignity. Bangladeshis are real fighters. They are frequently uprooted from one location by a natural disaster but within a year they relocate themselves elsewhere. They have fought well against nature and are on the verge of winning the battle against hunger. In this brave effort, they have received much help from national and international government and non-government organizations. The USA, particularly, has given large development funds as grants and loans. In addition to monetary aid, Bangladesh has also received considerable food aid, which has helped immensely in lifting food supply high enough to meet the effective demand.

Problems and characteristics

Bangladesh is fighting against heavy odds to produce enough food for its entire population. First, its geographical location, at the head of the Bay of Bengal and in the deltaic plains of the mighty Ganga and Brahmaputra, makes it one of the most precarious regions in the world. It is constantly under threat of floods, erosion, cyclones, and tidal waves of great ferocity. Second, there is an acute shortage of food-producing land and there is virtually no scope for its expansion. The land-people ratio is continually declining. It is worse than in China, Japan, and India. Due to the acute shortage of land, farmers take great risks in cultivating temporary river islands and areas prone to deep flooding. Third, there is great inequality in the distribution of income-earning resources, particularly land. More than 70 percent of the agricultural holdings are less than 2.5 acres in size, while 10 percent of the big landowners own 50 percent of the farmland. Therefore, a large proportion of the population is unemployed or underemployed, and makes little contribution to the generation of national wealth. Fourth, in the absence of a strong and well developed industrial sector, the purchased inputs required for food production are in short supply. Also, the growing population continues to be absorbed in agriculture.

The large and rapidly growing population makes the task of achieving self-sufficiency in food even more difficult. Nevertheless, it provides an abundant supply of labour and has made agriculture highly labour-intensive. Although landlessness is increasing, there is no evidence that this is due to population growth. The incidence of landlessness is more in the less densely populated western districts. Even the incidence of tenancy, which is often attributed to rapid population growth, is remarkably low. The agricultural landscape is overwhelmingly dominated by rice cultivation on small and fragmented holdings. The crop pattern changed significantly over the last two decades. Despite practically no change in the cultivated area, the area under rice increased by 12 percent. The area under *Boro* rice and wheat, both winter crops, increased most prominently. In 1972 *Boro* rice was the second-ranking crop in only one district but in 1992 it occupied second rank in several districts. The area under fruits and vegetables also increased quite considerably during the period. Quite understandably, the area under cash crops did not increase much during the period.

Crop regions also display significant change in the number of crops in each region. For example, three-crop combination regions occupied more districts in the final year than in the base year, indicating some increase in the spatial diversification of agriculture.

Achievements

Looking at the achievements of Bangladesh during the last two decades, no one can say that it is fighting a losing battle. Considering the strong 'environmental opposition' that Bangladesh faces, its achievements during the last two decades are remarkable indeed.

Despite declining land per agricultural worker, food producing capacity has continued to increase over time, the major contributors being multiple cropping and higher acre yields. During the two decades from 1972-73 to 1991-92, foodgrain production in Bangladesh increased at an annual rate of almost 4 percent, which was far greater than the population growth rate. In the same period rice production increased at an annual rate of 3.84 percent. The increase in rice production was almost entirely from increases in cropping intensity and yield per acre. The cropping intensity during the two decades increased from 142 to 172, and yield per acre of all rice varieties increased from 964 to 1419 lbs per acre. The yield per acre of rice increased by 47.2 percent in twenty years. In the 1980s, the increase in the per acre rice yield in Bangladesh was so large that it made an impact on the average rice yield of Asia. This impressive increase in rice yields was the result of large investment in water control, HYRVs, fertilizers, and agricultural research. During the same period, the increase in average wheat yields was even greater, but the contribution of wheat to the food supply was small because of the small acreage relative to rice. The consumption of foodgrains is beginning to increase in low income groups and declining in the high income groups. The increase in non-cereal foods such as fruits, vegetables, fish, meat, milk, and sugar also made a significant contribution to food supply. The consumption of fish and vegetables has been increasing in all income groups. Nevertheless, 2/3 of the protein intake still comes from cereals and only 1/3 from fish, pulses, and vegetables. One can, therefore, conclude that the food supply in Bangladesh during the two decades not only increased in quantity but also in quality. It is most satisfying to know that these improvements were not confined only to the average diet but that they trickled down to the diet of the low income households as well.

The three-year average domestic production of 10 major food items (rice, wheat, *masur*, gram, brinjal, potatoes, bananas, mangoes, jackfruit, and fish) supplied 2,132 calories per head per day, which was 7 percent above the MRDCR. Largely due to this increase in domestic food supply, the extent of hunger in Bangladesh declined from 83 percent to 47 percent of the total population. This is well supported by a significant decline in infant mortality. The domestic food supply is now enough to provide more than 2000 calories to each consumption unit. Therefore, the persistence of hunger is more a problem of maldistribution than of inadequate food supply. The bulk of this change in the extent of hunger is accounted for by the food exchange ratio of wages and per capita availability of food from domestic production. In the regression model used, these two variables together account for 80 percent of the variation in the extent of hunger over time.

The achievements recorded above clearly reveal that the domestic food supply in Bangladesh has increased faster than population and the Malthusian dragon has been nearly slain even in Bangladesh. This is demonstrated by increases not only in total production but also in land and labor productivities. Increases in food supply and some genuine efforts to protect food exchange entitlements of the poor have generated a consistent decline in hunger. The experience of Bangladesh supports the view that hunger is caused not by lack of resources but by flaws in socio-economic systems (Uvin 1994).

Prospects

In the last two decades, food supply increased entirely as a result of increases in multiple cropping and per acre yields of food crops. This implies that in the future too additional food must come from increases in these two. The question, therefore, arises: what are the prospects for further increasing multiple cropping and acre yields?

At present the average cropping intensity index for Bangladesh is 172, which is quite high, but it can be increased further. We have shown in Chapter 5 that cropping intensity has continued to increase with increasing population density over time. There is also a significant but modest correlation between the distribution patterns of cropping intensity and population density over space at one point in time. But there is no significant regional correlation between the growth rates of the two variables. This means that cropping intensity is no longer continuing to increase in the densely populated districts, i.e., it is not responding to further population growth. To explain this situation we have presented a regional theory of cropping intensity. The theory states that in the densely populated regions cropping intensity, in terms of the frequency of cultivation, after reaching a certain maximum ceases to respond to population growth. After this point, motivated by market forces, it begins to flow over into less densely populated regions. Therefore, it may be argued that in the future cropping intensity may not increase very much in the densely populated central and southeastern districts of Bangladesh, but there is still ample scope for its increase in the relatively less populated western and northern districts. In some regions, where the cropping pattern is dominated by short duration food crops, the cropping intensity can theoretically reach an index value of 300. The scope for increasing cropping intensity has increased enormously in recent years due to rapid spread of the early maturing HYRVs and fertilizer use.

Similarly, there is considerable scope for further increasing acre yields of rice and wheat, because they are still below several tropical Asian countries such as Indonesia, Malaysia, South China, and Taiwan, and also below the Asian average. Comparing the current acre yield of clean rice with a rather modest potential target of 2000 lbs per acre suggests that rice yields can be raised by at least 30 percent above the present level. As has been the case during the last two decades, the major source of future growth in acre yields will be further expansion of HYRVs and HYVs of wheat and other crops. This, of course, will require further expansion of irrigation and fertilizer use. There is considerable scope for expansion of both. A 30 percent increase in the average crop yields will make Bangladesh more than self-sufficient, and leave a large surplus for meeting additional demand due to population increases and for exports. Assuming that the food supply can be increased by 30 percent, the domestic production should be able to feed the growing population for the next 15 years or so, if the population continues to grow at the present rate. But the indications are that the population growth is slowing down and it may become stabilised in the next 15 or 20 years. Hence, there are good prospects that widespread deaths due to starvation may be avoided in Bangladesh. The flood control plan that is now under way will further help increase food supply and provide greater food security.

Further, plant scientists are continually working on the development of new rice varieties and have, in fact, announced the development of a new rice that will produce a lot more than the present varieties and will be more resistant to diseases. Some new varieties may be more resistant to droughts. Hence, it is entirely possible that the food supply potential in Bangladesh, in the near future, may exceed the 30 percent limit arrived at in this study.

Policy issues

The unfavourable people-resource ratio and the vulnerable geographical location of Bangladesh have prompted some people to say that Bangladesh cannot be a rich country. Perhaps it may be true, but there are several rich countries where the ratio is just as bad, such as the Netherlands, Japan, Denmark, and Singapore. But these are not agrarian economies. Therefore, it would be more appropriate to say that Bangladesh cannot expect to be a rich country without the development of a substantial manufacturing sector. In the context of food, one can say that Bangladesh cannot be a major food surplus country and can never reach the dietary standards of the rich western countries. But that is neither necessary nor desirable. If Bangladesh can attain self-sufficiency in its basic food requirements and produce a small surplus for building reserve stocks, that will be a great achievement. Bangladesh has the will and capacity to eradicate hunger and to provide the basic needs of all its people. But for doing that it may have to build a larger manufacturing sector in order to take away some population pressure from agricultural land, to generate foreign exchange for purchasing capital goods, and to provide support for modern agriculture. But these are broader issues of development and outside the scope of this study. Therefore, we will focus attention only on hunger eradication policies.

As far back as we go in history there always was some hunger in societies, just as continues to be even in the richest societies today (Kate and Milman 1990, Brown 1987). Therefore, in Bangladesh too some hunger may persist indefinitely, unless restrictions on ownership of resources required to produce or buy food are completely removed (Hossain 1994). But that is unlikely to happen. All that can be expected to happen is the reduction of hunger to a minimum level.

The policies to reduce hunger to a minimum level must be focused on identifying the causes of hunger and then trying to defuse their effect on hunger. In Bangladesh, hunger is caused by a combination of inadequate and unstable food supply, inequality in the ownership of resources required to produce or buy food, and inadequate public action for entitlement protection of the poor. The policies to reduce hunger and undernutrition must be focused on all these three issues simultaneously.

Policies to increase food supply

It is often argued that in the densely populated agrarian economies, where there is an acute shortage of arable land, replacement of foodgrains by high value labour-intensive food and non-food export crops such as fruits, vegetables, and flowers would be more effective in the fight against hunger and poverty (Kennedy and Cogill 1987, Bonis and Hoddad 1990). The proponents of this view say that by doing this peasant farmers on their small holdings will earn more income per acre and will be able to buy more food from the world market than they can produce. It may sound good in theory but is not always so in practice. The countries who adopt such a scheme may become too dependent on the nations that import their perishable food and supply them with foodgrains in return, and may not be able to confront them when necessary on any important issues. They may run the risk of losing their freedom to decide for themselves what ideologies and foreign policies to choose and support. They may become politically very vulnerable, and in the event of opposing the major policies of the countries they buy their food from they may run the risk of facing trade embargoes and bans that may cause widespread hunger. Moreover, if many countries start producing fruits, vegetable, and flowers, the prices of these items will fall relative to manufactured goods and even foodgrains.

Salma and Warr (1994) believe that Bangladesh will be better off by removing all restrictions on foodgrain imports. They think that complete liberalization of foodgrain imports will increase food supply, exports in general, and employment, and reduce prices. It may be a good policy for countries having a strong manufacturing sector such as Japan, Korea, and Singapore in Asia, and several countries in Europe. But even these countries, who have plenty of foreign exchange to buy any amount of food from anywhere in the world, are strongly opposed to such a policy. It is beyond our comprehension how a country like Bangladesh, which has practically no exportable natural resources and only an insignificant manufacturing sector, can successfully adopt such a policy.

The commendable success of Bangladesh in increasing food supply is an indication that the existing policies are in the right direction and proving effective. The drive to achieve self-sufficiency in basic food is essential for a country like Bangladesh. The country has almost reached the goal through widespread adoption of new technology (water, fertilizer, and seed technology) and there is still considerable scope for its further expansion. All that is required is to make the existing policies more effective for the promotion of the new technology. For example, in some regions the adoption of new technology has been slow because of poor infrastructure (Ahmad 1989). Therefore, the policy to increase food supply further must concentrate more on the construction of roads, bridges, irrigation channels, vertical irrigation tanks, land embankments, grain drying pans, depots for the sale of subsidised inputs, and storage facilities, and development of banks and markets. Furthermore, domestic production of fertilizers, insecticides, and irrigation equipment should receive a high priority in industrial development policy. The manufacturing of agricultural inputs must be encouraged even if it has to be based on some imported raw materials. The existing policy of giving higher priority to the promotion of dry season winter crops is again in the right direction, because winter crops are less vulnerable to damage from natural disasters. Both *Boro* rice and wheat have made important contributions to increasing food supply. Now attention should be given to other winter crops that require less water such as gram, barley, lentils, and oil seeds. There is always a ready demand for oil seeds in the world market, and therefore any surplus can be easily exported. For gram and barley there is considerable demand in both domestic and international markets, for human consumption and livestock feed.

Although it is true that fertilizer subsidies were mainly helping the big farmers, the government policy to phase them out is not in the right direction. It will adversely affect the small farmers. To further encourage the spread of HYV food crops, the supply of subsidised inputs to small farmers must continue. The promotion of new technology on small farms is most desirable, because the small farmers, who often suffer from hunger, will be directly benefited by increased production. Small scale production involves more people and therefore benefits will be distributed to a larger section of the poor or food poor population (Stamp 1977). It appears that water control is the key factor for increasing food supply in Bangladesh, and it has rightly received a high priority in public policy, particularly since independence. At present, the area under irrigation and flood control is only 30 and 15 percent of the cultivated area respectively, but it can be increased to 60 and 65 percent. From the mid-1970s the policy shifted in favour of small scale irrigation projects such as deep and shallow tube-wells. The latter proved particularly effective, and their number increased from 4,000 in 1975 to about 80,000 in 1991. The shallow tube-wells have contributed immensely to increases in food supply. Much of the surface water still goes to waste, and it can be collected in vertical concrete tanks to provide additional irrigation for winter crops and at the same time prevent some areas from flooding in summer. The shift in irrigation policy is helping to increase output on small farms. The greater success of new technology on large farms may perhaps lead to mechanization but on small farms it may create demand for hired labour. Human labour, of course, may be more expensive than machines, but society is better off when more people are employed (Foster 1992). Therefore, subsidizing labour costs on both large and small farms will be an effective measure to increase food supply and reduce hunger.

Efforts more recently to increase fruits, vegetables, and fish have ushered in a new dimension in food policy in Bangladesh, and this is already causing a welcome change in food consumption patterns of the rich as well as the poor.

Environmental impact of the new technology

The declining yields of HYRVs are serious and demand the urgent attention of the policy makers in Bangladesh. It is a warning that HYRVs may make a greatly curtailed contribution to food supply in the near future. The declining yields of HYRVs are probably due to high frequency of cropping and greatly increased use of fertilizers. Chemical fertilizers increase immediate crop yields but their prolonged use damages the soil structure, because the organic matter of the soil is not replenished. Soil gradually loses its porosity and becomes less responsive to fertilizers. The declining HYRVs in Bangladesh may be indicating the negative impact of chemical fertilizers.

Although at present fertilizer consumption per hectare in Bangladesh is only 3 percent of that of Japan, 8 percent of that of the USA, and 16 percent of that of the Asian average, one cannot completely ignore the agronomic and environmental problems caused by prolonged and excessive use of chemical fertilizers (Biswas 1994). In the temperate countries, uninterrupted use of chemical fertilizers may not do as much damage to soils as in the tropical and sub-tropical climates. In the USA and Japan, for example, soil is not cultivated for 4 to 5 months because temperatures are too low for plant growth. Hence, the soil gets time for rejuvenation. But in a country like Bangladesh, where the soil is cultivated throughout the year for crop production, the damage to soil from continuous use of chemical fertilizers is bound to be much greater. Hence, one cannot support, without reservations, the continuation of the present policy of increasing food supply through indefinite expansion of seed-water-fertilizer technology. Within the next few years, when self-sufficiency is more firmly established, the policy makers in Bangladesh must begin to implement some modifications in the policy to make food supply more sustainable.

An important aspect of the food policy must be concerned with the restoration of soil fertility in order to maintain the established positive trend in the food supply. This may best be done by growing HYRVs and other HYV crops within an improved mixed farming system. In this system crops and animals are raised in close proximity, each supporting the other. Crop residue and fodder crops supply animal feed, and animals in return supply draft power and manure for the crops in addition to milk and meat. This was the normal practice in Bangladesh not very long ago and can be revived with some improvements. Cereals may be rotated with legumes and vegetables. Legumes are already important in the cropping pattern and the common diet of the people in Bangladesh. Legumes can fix up to 200 lbs of nitrogen per acre and thereby reduce the need for chemical fertilizers (Owen 1980). The change has already started even in America where chemical farming first began. Some California rice farmers on the floodplains of rivers, using only organic manure, are producing four to five time more rice per acre than farmers growing HYRVs in Bangladesh (Klinkenborg 1995). They save at least $100 per acre in costs, compared with farmers using chemical fertilizers, and get more income because they produce more. Substitutes for inorganic nitrogenous fertilizers are being tried in several rice growing regions and are proving successful. An experiment conducted by Pandey et al. (1995) showed that using 100 kg of nitrogen per hectare gave initially 6 tons of rice per hectare but the yield then steadily declined over time. But using 60 kg of nitrogen per hectare with green manuring and some farmyard manure produced 6.8 tons of rice per hectare, a level which was maintained for several years. The second method was somewhat dearer, but the higher cost was more than compensated for by higher yields and maintenance of soil fertility. Bar and Dhillon (1994) found that the application of green manuring and farmyard manure not only increase rice yields but also improves the soil structure — its organic carbon content. A return to organic farming will be gradual. In Bangladesh, perhaps, for a start, chemical fertilizers can be supplemented with animal manure in the ratio of 80 and 20 percent respectively. As the system gets established the quantity of chemical fertilizers may be gradually reduced and that of organic manure increased.

The revival of a crop-rotation-organic system of food production will not be difficult, because in Bangladesh it was the norm not very long ago. A food supply system based on crop rotation and organic manure is just as productive as that based on chemicals, if not more productive, and is more sustainable.

Continuing research on new rice varieties provides further promise for the eradication of hunger in the near future even for the growing population. Plant genetic engineers at the IRRI are striving to produce new rice varieties that will produce much higher yields than the HYRVs cultivated at present and will have a higher grain to straw ratio. They have already announced the development of a new rice that holds the promise of a dramatic increase in world rice production. The miracle rice, as yet unnamed, will become a reality by the end of the century (IRRI 1993). It is expected to give 30 percent higher yield than the varieties presently cultivated. The new rice plant will have 60 percent grain and 40 percent straw. Research at the IRRI and its numerous national branches is also quite advanced on developing rice varieties that will be more tolerant to disease, temperatures, and droughts. Hence, the potential yields of these new varieties may be far greater than the yield of those cultivated at present.

However, a matter of serious concern that has surfaced recently is that the HYVs of rice and wheat provide enough calories but are poor in some essential micronutrients such as iron and zinc and vitamins (*New Scientist* 1996). Therefore, in some regions where food supply and average calorie intake have increased due to HYVs of foodgrains, diseases associated with mineral and vitamin deficiencies have increased. This has drawn the attention of the plant scientists to the development of new strains of rice and wheat that are both rich in minerals and vitamins and also high yielding. The development of such strains is entirely possible because some major genes in plants have a greater ability to draw micronutrients from the soil, for example, the genes in tomatoes, soya beans, and maize draw more iron from the soil than other crop plants. The research should now be focused on fixing such genes in rice and wheat, but that, of course, will take a long time. The immediate action should be to educate and encourage people to use with rice more leafy vegetables and beans that are cheap and are found in great abundance in the tropical and semi-tropical regions.

In Bangladesh this dietary problem does not appear to be so serious, because the average consumption of vegetables, fruits, and fish has been increasing over time in all income groups. Nevertheless, a nutrition program should be seriously launched to encourage people to eat more green leafy vegetables, beans, and fruits. Several of these food items are quite cheap and often can be collected free of cost from public and unused private land.

Policies to reduce instability in food supply

Food supply is subject to annual, seasonal, and regional fluctuations everywhere and especially so in Bangladesh. During the reference period the average coefficient of variation for cereals was 19.16, which remained largely unchanged. However, individual cereals recorded considerable changes in variability. For example, the coefficient of variation for the total production of *Aman* and *Aus* declined slightly but that for *Boro* increased quite significantly. In general, the instability of production from HYVs was higher than the instability of total production of each variety of rice. The output of rain-fed crops, like *Aman* and *Aus*, became slightly more stable during the period, perhaps due to the benefits from the flood control programs. It appears that the rain-fed varieties of rice have become more adapted to their environment and are able to resist departures from normal better than the irrigated crops. The total production instability is the lowest for *Aman* and the highest for *Boro*. This may be because a very high percentage of *Boro* rice is under the HYVs relative to *Aman*. The instability in wheat production was high in the 1970s but declined slightly in the 1980s as the crop became more established. It is important to note that as the HYRVs are helping to increase food supply they are also likely to make it more unstable. This is because HYVs are less tolerant to droughts and floods and more prone to diseases.

It is these fluctuations in supply that threaten food security and often trigger the mechanism that leads to entitlement failure (Gommes 1993). Therefore, part of the food policy must be aimed at reducing instability in food supply. While Bangladesh can do practically nothing to reduce the damaging effects of cyclones and sea waves on food production, it can certainly minimize the effects of floods and droughts, if suitable action is taken. The flood protection program has received a high priority and is progressing well. It involves building embankments on both banks of all major rivers, dredging of river beds where they are shallow, and storage of water for dry season crops. These programs will considerably reduce crop damage. Reforestation all along the northern borders and even planting fruit trees along the boundaries of relatively bigger rice fields will reduce the damage caused by floods. Reforestation may take away some land from food production but the loss may be more than compensated for by land saved from erosion and additional food from tree crops.

Much more could be done in reducing crop damage from droughts. Further expansion of irrigation facilities, for which there is plenty of scope in Bangladesh, is required to minimize damage from droughts. The collection of flood waters in vertical concrete tanks is a real possibility that needs serious consideration.

Also, public investment in storage of foodgrains for the lean years is yet another important requirement that must be undertaken more seriously than at present. Adequate reserve stocks must be built up so that Bangladesh does not have to depend upon the international community for food aid after every natural disaster. This is necessary for building the self esteem of the people.

No matter how much is done to reduce the effect of climate on the food supply, the supply will always suffer from some instability. Therefore, while everything possible must be done to reduce the effect of climate on food production, it is also essential to build up reserve foodgrain stocks and systems of storing them.

Our analysis clearly shows that no matter how much food supply is increased and stabilized, it may still not reach a high proportion of the hungry population. To make food available to them, determined efforts will have to be made to protect and improve their food entitlements. Policies in this direction are somewhat lacking in Bangladesh. The present government policy favours the urbanites, but the majority of the hungry live in the rural areas (Khan and Hossain 1989). The urban bias in policy incurs a welfare loss of more than 12 billion Takas annually to the rural poor and depresses local production (Hossain 1994). This is regarded by some researchers as the major cause of chronic food shortage in the country. The majority of existing policies such as statutory rationing, employment creation in the public sector, public expenditure on education, and subsidies on inputs have not helped the poor. There are only a few policies such as the Food for Work Program, Credit for the Rural Poor by the Grameen Bank, and Destitute Group Feeding that have directly helped the poor.

There is an urgent need for government policies in this area to be substantially modified in order to help the poor and reduce hunger. The statutory rationing and modified rationing schemes must be changed to benefit only the poor. Similarly just as the government creates employment in the public sector for the benefit of the urban population it must also create more employment opportunities in the rural areas for the landless and the small farmers. Re-establishment of some cottage and labour-intensive processing industries will be most helpful. Such opportunities will also have a positive impact on agricultural wages, particularly during the slack agricultural months. There is no doubt that the food exchange ratio of the agricultural wages has increased over time, but they must rise further to allow some savings for dormant periods, when there is little or no work available to agricultural workers.

Although the question is debatable, it is our view, hunger can be reduced further by implementing an effective land reform policy, leading to some redistribution of land. Concentration of land in a few hands is an obstacle to the spread of new agricultural technology, which has been a key factor in increasing food supply in Bangladesh. There is unmistakeable evidence that not only productivity but also the diffusion of new technology are higher on small farms. There is also the danger that increased profits derived from new technology on large farms may encourage owners to evict tenant farmers from their land and have it cultivated by hired labour. This will further increase inequality and push more people below the poverty line. Hence, it is essential that some kind of land reform policy be effectively implemented in Bangladesh.

Bibliography

Abdullah, A. (1976), 'Land reform and agrarian change in Bangladesh', *Bangladesh Development Studies* , Vol. 4, No. 4, October.

Abdullah, M. and Wheeler, E. F. (1985), 'Seasonal variations and intra-household distribution of food in a Bangladesh village', *American Journal of Clinical Nutrition*, Vol. 41, No. 6, June.

Abedin, J. and Bose, G.K. (1988), 'Farm size and productivity differences — a decomposition analysis', *Bangladesh Development Studies*, Vol. 16, No. 3, September.

Achaya, K.T. (1983), 'RDAs: their limitations and applications', *Economic and Political Weekly*, Vol. 18, No. 15, April.

ADAB (1983), *Food Aid to Bangladesh*. Canberra: Australian Government Publication Service.

_____ (1981), *Regional Disaster Preparedness Seminar*. Canberra. Australian Government Publication Service.

Ahmad, A.U., Khan, A.H., and Sampath, R.K. (1991), 'Poverty in Bangladesh: measurement, decomposition, and inter-temporal comparison', *Journal of Development Studies*, Vol. 27, No. 4, July.

Ahamd, R. (1987),'A structural perspective of farm and non-farm households in Bangladesh', *Bangladesh Development Studies*, Vol. 15, No.2, June.

_____ (1989), *Making Rural Infrastructure a Priority*. Research Report No. 11, Washington, DC: International Food Policy Research Institute.

Ahluwalia, M.S. (1978), 'Rural poverty and agricultural performance', *Journal of Development Studies*, Vol. 14, No. 2, April.

_____ (1985), 'Rural poverty, agricultural production, and prices: a re-examination, in Mellor, J. W. and Desai, G. (eds), *Agricultural Change and Rural Poverty*. Baltimore: Johns Hopkins Press.

Alam, S. (1992), 'Have supply responses increased for major crops in Bangladesh ?', *Bangladesh Development Studies*, Vol. 20, No. 1, March.

Alauddin, M. and Tisdell, C. (1987), 'Trends and projections in Bangladesh food production: an alternative viewpoint', *Food Policy*, Vol. 12, No. 4, October.

Ali, A. M.S. and Turner, II, B. L. (1990), *Agricultural Stagnation or Growth: Change in Six Villages in Bangladesh 1950-1985*. Clark University: Unpublished Manuscript.

Anthes, R. A. (1981), *Tropical Cyclones: Their Evolution, Structure, and Effects*. Boston: American Meteorological Society.

Antle, J. M. (1983), 'Infrastructure and aggregate agricultural productivity: International evidence', *Economic Development and Cultural Change*, Vol. 31, No. 3, April.

Arnon, I. (1987), *Modernization of Agriculture in Developing Countries: Resources, Potentials, and Problems*. New York: John Wiley and Sons.

Asaduzzaman, M. and Huddleston, B. (1983), 'An evaluation of food for work program', *Bangladesh Development Studies*, Vol. 11, Nos. 1&2, January & April.

Ayoob, M., Gupta, A., Khan, A. and Deshpande, G. P. (1971), *Bangladesh: A Struggle for Nationhood*. New Delhi: Vikas Publication.

Bairagi, R. (1986), 'Food crisis, nutritional status, and female children in Bangladesh', *Population and Development Review*, Vol. 12, Nos.1-2, Supplement, June.

Banik, A. (1990), 'Changes in agrarian structure in Bangladesh: 1960-1984', *Bangladesh Development Studies*, Vol. 18, No. 4, October.

Baliscan, A. M. (1993), 'Agricultural growth, landlessness, off-farm employment, and rural poverty in the Philippines', *Economic Development and Cultural Change*, Vol. 41, No. 3, April.

Bar, B. S. and Dhillon, N. S. (1994), 'Effects of farmyard manure application on yield and soil fertility in rice and wheat rotation', *International Rice Research Notes*, Vol. 19, No.2, April.

Bardhan, P.K. (1973), 'On the incidence of poverty in rural India of the sixties', *Economic and Political Weekly*, Vol. 8, Annual Number, February.

Barlowe, R. (1972), *Land Economics*. Englewood Cliffs: Prentice Hall.

Barrow, C.J. (1991), *Land Degradation*. Cambridge: Cambridge University Press.

Barrow, E. M. (1993), 'Geographical complexities of detailed impact assessment for Ganges, Brahamaputra, and Meghna delta of Bangladesh', in Warrick, R. A. and Wigley, T.M.L. (eds.), *Climate and Seasonal Change*. Cambridge: Cambridge University Press.

Basehart, W. (1973), 'Cultivation intensity, settlement patterns, and homestead farms among the Matengo of Tanzania', *Ethnology*, Vol. 12, No. 1, January.

Battuta, I. (1958), *Travels of Ibn Battuta* (English Translation by A. Constable). Cambridge University Press.

Bautista, R. M. (1988), 'Agricultural growth as a development strategy for the Philippines', *Philippines Economic Journal*, Vol. 27, No. 1, January.

Bengoa, J.M. (1972), 'Nutritional significance of mortality statistics', in *Proceedings of the Third Western Hemisphere Nutrition Congress.* New York: Futura.

Bennet, J. (1987), *Hunger Machine.* Cambridge: Polity Press.

Bera, A. K. and Kelly, T. G. (1990), 'Adoption of high yielding rice varieties in Bangladesh: an econometric analysis', *Journal of Development Economics*, Vol. 33, No. 2, October.

Bernier, F. (1891, Reprinted 1968), *Trends in Moughal Empire, AD 1656-1688.* Delhi: S. Chand and Co.

Bhattacharya, N., Chatterjee, G.S., and Pal, P. (1988), 'Variations in level of living in regions and special groups in rural India', in Srinivasan, T. N. and Bardhan, P. K., *Rural Poverty in South Asia.* New York: Columbia University Press.

Bilsborrow, R. E. (1987), 'Population pressure and agricultural development in developing countries: a conceptual framework and recent evidence', *World Development,* Vol. 15, No. 2, February.

Biswas, M. (1994), 'Nutrition, food production, and environment', in Biswas, M. and Gabar, M. (eds), *Nutrition in the Nineties.* Delhi: Oxford University Press.

Blyn, G. (1966), *Agricultural Trends in India: Output, Availability and Productivity.* Philadelphia: University of Pennsylvania Press.

Bonis, H. E. and Haddad, L. (1990), The Effects of Agricultural Commercialization on Land Tenure, Household Resource Allocations, and Nutrition in Philippines. Research Report No. 79, Washington, D.C.: International Food Policy Research Institute.

Booth, A. (1988), *Agricultural Development in Indonesia,* Sydney: Allen and Unwin.

Boserup, E. (1965, *Conditions of Agricultural Growth: The Economics of Agrarian Change Under Population Pressure.* London: George Allen and Unwin.

_____ (1975), 'The impact of population growth on agricultural output', *Quarterly Journal of Economics* , Vol. 89, No. 2, April.

_____ (1981), *Population and Technology .* Oxford: Basil Blackwell.

_____ (1990), *Economic and Demographic Relationships in Development.* Baltimore: Johns Hopkins University Press.

Boyce, J.K. (1987), *Agrarian Impasse in Bengal.* Oxford: Oxford University Press.

Bradley, P.N. and Carter, S. E. (1989), 'Food production, distribution, and hunger', in Jonhston, R. J. and Taylor, P. J. (eds.), *A World in Crisis: Geographical Perspectives.* Cambridge: Basil Blackwell.

Brammer, H. (1990), 'Floods in Bangladesh 1', *The Geographical Journal,* Vol. 156, No. 1, March.

_____ , 'Floods in Bangladesh 2', *The Geographical Journal,* Vol. 156, No. 2, July.

Brookfield, H. (1962), 'Local study and comparative method: an example from Central New Guinea', *Annals of the Association of American Geographer* , Vol. 52, No. 1, March.

_____ (1972), 'Intensification and disintensification of Pacific agriculture', *Pacific View Point*, Vol.13, No.1, May.

_____ *et al.* (1990), 'Borneo and Malaya Penninsula', in Turner , B.L. *et al.* (eds), *The Earth as Transformed by Human Action.* Cambridge: Cambridge University Press.

Brown, D. (1971), *Agricultural Development in India's Districts.* Cambridge, Mass.: Harvard University Press.

Brown, J. L.(1987), 'Hunger in the USA', *Scientific Amrican*, Vol. 256, No. 2, February.

Brown, P. and Podolesky, A. (1976), 'Popultion density, agricultural intensity, land tenure, and group size in New Guinea Highlands', *Ethnology* , Vol. 15, No. 3, July.

Butzar, Karl W. (1990), 'The realm of cultural human ecology: adoption and change in historical perspective', in Turner, B. L. *et al.* (eds), *The Earth as Transformed by Human Action.* Cambridge: Cambridge University Press.

Carlstein, T. (1982), *Time, Resources, Society, and Ecology: on the Capacity for Human Interaction in Space and Time.* London: George Allen and Unwin.

Chakravarti, A.K. (1970), 'Foodgrain Sufficiency Patterns in India', *Geographical Review*, Vol. 60, No. 2, April.

_____ (1974), 'Regional preference for food: some aspects of food habits patterns in India', *The Canadian Geographer*, Vol. 18, No. 4, December.

_____ (1976), 'The impact of high yielding varieties program on food-grain production in India', *Canadian Geographer*, Vol. 20, No. 2, April.

Chakravarty, S. (1984), 'Power structure and agricultural productivity', in Desai, M., Rudolph, S. H., and Rudra, A. (eds.), *Agrarian Power and Agricultural Productivity in South Asia.* Berkeley: University of California Press.

Chang, Jen-Hu (1968), 'The agricultural potential of the humid tropics', *Geographical Review*, Vol. 58, No. 2, April.

Chatfield, R. (1808), *An Historical Review of the Commercial, Political, and Moral Status of Hindoostan.* London: J. M. Richardson.

Chaudhary, M.K. and Anjea, D.R. (1991), 'Impact of Green revolution on long term sustainability of land and water resources in Haryana', *Indian Journal of Agricultural Economics*, Vol. 46, No. 3, July.

Chaudhury, R.H. (1981), 'Population pressure and agricultural productivity', *Bangladesh Development Studies*, Vol. 9, No. 1, March.

_____ (1989), 'Population pressure and its effects on changes in agrarian structure and productivity in rural Bangladesh', In Garry Rodgers (ed.) *Population Growth and Poverty in Rural South Asia.* New Delhi: Sage Publication.

Chen, L.C. and Chaudhury, R.H. (1975),'Demographic change and food production', *Population and Development Review* , Vol. 1, No.1, March.

Chen, L. C.; Huq, E.; and D'Souza, S. (1981), 'Sex bias in the family allocation of food and health care in rural Bangladesh', *Population and Development Review*, Vol. 7, No. 1, March.

Chiras, D.D. (1991), *Environmental Science— Action for a Sustainable Future*. Redwood City: California, The Benjamin Publishing Co.

Chowdhury, N. (1988), 'Accounting for subsidized food resources distributed in statutory rationing in Bangladesh', *Bangladesh Development Studies*, Vol. 16, No. 4, December.

———— (1987), 'Seasonality of foodgrain prices and procurement program in Bangladesh since liberation: an exploratory study', *Bangladesh Development Studies*, Vol. 15, No.1, March.

Chowdhury, S. R. (1972), *The Genesis of Bangladesh*. London: Asia Publishing House.

Clark, C. (1957), *Conditions of Economic Progress*. London: Macmillan.

Clarke, W.C. (1966), 'From extensive to intensive cultivation: a succession from New Guinea', *Ethnology*, Vol. 5, No. 4, October.

Coale, A. J. and Hoover, E. M. (1958), *Population Growth and Economic Development in Low Income Countries*. Princeton: Princeton University Press.

Cobb, C. E. Jr.(1993), 'When the water comes', *National Geographic*, Vol. 183, No. 6, June.

Coppock, J. T. (1966), *An Agricultural Atlas of England and Wales*. London: Faber and Co.

Crosson, P. (1982), *The Cropland Crisis: Myth or Reality*. Baltimore: Johns Hopkins Press.

Curry, B. (1984), 'Fragile mountains or fragile theory', *Agricultural Development Agencies in Bangladesh, News*, Vol. 6, No. 11, November.

Dandekar, V.M. (1981), 'On measurement of poverty', *Economic and Political Weekly*, Vol. 16, No. 30, July.

———— and Rath, N. (1971), *Poverty in India: Dimensions and Trends*. Poona: Indian School of Political Economy.

Dasgupta, Monica (1987), 'Informal security mechanism and population retention in rural India', *Economic Development and Cultural Change*, Vol. 36, No. 1, October.

Dasgupta, P. and Ray, D. (1990), 'Adapting to undernuourishment: the biological evidence and its implications', in Dreze, J. and Sen, A. (eds.), *The Political Economy of Hunger*. Oxford: Clarendon Press.

———— (1986), 'Inequality as a determinant of malnutrition and unemployment: Theory', *Economic Journal*, Vol. 96, No. 384, December.

Dayal, E. (1967), 'Crop combination regions: A case study of the Punjab Plains', *Tijdschrift voor Econ. En Soc. Geografie*, Vol. 58, No. 1, January.

_____ (1974), 'The present pertinence of Von Thunen theory in an advance economy: a case of southeast Australia', *Proceedings of the International Geographical Union Regional Conference and Eight New Zealand Geography Conference*, Palmerston North: New Zealand.

_____ (1977), 'Impact of irrigation expansion on multiple cropping in India', *Tijdschrift voor Economische en Sociale Geografi e*, Vol. 68, No. 2, March.

_____ (1984), 'Agricultural productivity in India: A spatial analysis', *Annals Association of American Geographers* , Vol. 74, No. 1, March.

_____ (1988), 'Nutritional wage over time and space in Bangladesh', *Canadian Geographer*, Vol. 32, No. 2, April.

_____ (1989), 'Land and labor productivity in Bangladesh agriculture', *Asian Profile* , Vol. 17, No. 4, August..

_____ (1990), 'Sources of labour productivity in Bangladesh agriculture', *GeoJournal*, Vol. 20, No. 3, March.

Desai, M. and Majumdar, D. (1970), 'A test of hypothesis of disguised unemployment', *Economica*, Vol. 37, Nos. 145-148 (no month).

Dixon, C. (1990), *Rural Development in the Third World*. London: Routledge.

Dreze, J. and Sen, A. (1989), *Hunger and Public Action*. Oxford: Clarendon Press.

Dutra de Oliveira, J., Dos Santos, J., and Desai, I. (1985), 'Commentry', in O. Burnser et al. (eds.), *Clinical Nutrition of the Young Child*. New York: Raven Press.

Dutta, K. K. (1936), *Studies in the Economy of Bengal Suba*. Calcutta: Calcutta University Press.

Eckholm, E.P. (1976), *Loosing Ground: Environmental Stress and the World Food Prospects*. New York: Norton.

Eder, J. F. (1977), 'Agricultural intensification and the returns to labor in the Philippines swidden system', *Pacific Viewpoint* , Vol. 18, No. 1, January.

Ehrlich, P.R. (1968), *The Population Bomb*. New York: Ballantine.

Ehrlich, P.R. et al. (1977), *Ecoscience*. San Francisco: W.H. Freeman and Co.

Ehrlich, P. R.; Ehrlich, A. H.; and Daily, G. C. (1993), 'Food security, population, and environment', *Population and Development Review*, Vol. 19, No. 1, March.

Evanson, R.E. and Y. Kisleve (1975), *Agricultural Rsearch and Productivity*. New Haven: Yale University Press.

FAO (1977), *The Fourth World Food Survey*. Rome.

_____ (1974), *Production Yearbook 1973*. Geneva.

_____ (1993), *Production Yearbook 1993*. Geneva.

Foster, P. (1992), *The World Food Problem*. Boulder: Lynne Rienner Publishers.

Geddes, A. (1937), 'The population of Bengal, its distribtution and changes: a contribution to geographical method', *Geographical Journal*, Vol. 89, No. 4, April.

Geertz, J. (1963), *Agricultural Involution; The Process of Ecological Change in Indonesia*. Berkeley: University of California Press.

Gill, G. J. (1983), 'Mechanical land preparation, productivity, and employment in

Gill, G. J. (1983), 'Mechanical land preparation, productivity, and employment in Bangladesh agriculture', *The Journal of Development Studies*, Vol. 19, No. 3, April.

Gillespie, S. and Mc Neill, G. (1992), *Food, Health, and Survival in India and Developing Countries*. New Delhi: Vikas Publications.

Gleave, M.B. and White, H.P. (1969), 'Population density and agricultural systems in West Africa.', in M. F. Thomas (ed.), *Environment and Land Use in West Africa*. London: Methuen.

Gommes, R. (1993), 'Current climate and population constraints on world agriculture', in Kaiser, H. M. and Drennen, T. E. (eds), *Agricultural Dimensions of Global Climate Change*. Delsay Beach: St. Lucie Press.

G. O. B. (1983), *The Second Five Year Plan*. Dhaka: Ministry of Finance and Planning.

———— (1985), *Upazila Statistics Vol. 1 (1979-80 to 1982-83)*. Dhaka: Bangladesh Bureau of Statistics.

———— (1986), *Census of Agriculture and Livestock*. Dhaka: Bangladesh Bureau of Statistics.

———— (1986), *Bangladesh Census of Agriculture and Livestock: 1 983-84*, Vol. 1, Dhaka: Bangladesh Bureau of Statistics.

———— (1987), *Yearbook of Agricultural Statistics 1985-86*. Dhaka: Bangladesh Bureau of Statistics.

———— (1988), *Statistical Yearbook 1987*. Dhaka: Bangladesh Bureau of Statistics.

———— (1991), *Report on Household Expenditure Survey, 1988-89*. Dhaka: Bangladesh Bureau of Statistics.

———— (1995), *Summary Report on Household Expenditure Survey 1991-92*. Dhaka: Bangladesh Bureau of Statistics.

———— (1982, 1984, 1988, 1992 and 1993), *Statistical Yearbook of Bangladesh*. Dhaka: Bangladesh Bureau of Statistics.

G. O. I. (1964), *Census of India 1961*. New Delhi: Manager of Publications.

Gopalan, C. et al. (1981), *Nutritive Value of Indian Foods*. Hyderabad: Indian Council of Medical Research.

———— (1983), 'Measurement of undernutrition', *Economic and Political Weekly*, Vol.18, No. 15, April.

Greenough, P. R. (1982), *Prosperity and Misery in Modern Bengal: The Famine of 1943-44*. New York: Oxford University

Grine, I. D. and Harrison, G. A. (1988), *Coping with Uncertainty in Food Supply*. Oxford: Clarendon Press.

Grigg, D. (1974), *The Agricultural Systems of the World: An Evolutionary Approach*. Cambridge: Cambridge University Press.

Grossman, D. (1984), 'Agricultural intensification and population in Northern Samaria: Changes in the olive-grain ratio', *Geografiska Annaler* (Series B, Human Geography), Vol. 66, No. 2(no month).

Habakuk, J. (1963), 'Population problems and European economic development in the late eighteenth and nineteenth century', *American Economic Review*, Vol. 53, No. 2, May.

Habib, I. (1963), *The Agrarian System of Mughal India*. Bombay: Asia Publishing House.

Hanson, H. and Norman, E. (1982), *Wheat in the Third World*. Boulder: Westview Press.

Haque, C. E. and Hossain, Z. (1988), 'River bank erosion in Bangladesh', *Geographical Review*, Vol. 78, No. 1, January.

Harris, B. (1990), 'Intra-family distribution of hunger in South Asia', in J. Dreze and A. Sen (eds.), *Poitical Economy of Hunger*, Vol. 1. Oxford: Oxford University Press.

Hayami, Y. and Ruttan, V.W. (1971), *Agricultural Development: An International Perspective*. Baltimore: Johns Hopkins University Press.

Hayami, Y. and Ruttan, W. (1985), *Agricultural Development: An International Perspective*. Baltimore: Johns Hopkins University Press.

Hossain, M. (1977), 'Farm size, tenancy, and land productivity: an analysis of farm level data in Bangladesh agriculture', *The Bangladesh Development Studies*, Vol. 5, No. 3, July.

_____ (1980), 'Foodgrain production in Bangladesh: Performance, potential, and constraints', *Bangladesh Development Studies*, Vol. 8, Nos. 1&2, January & June.

_____ (1984), 'Agricultural development in Bangladesh: a historical perspective', *Bangladesh Development Studies*, Vol. 12, No. 1, March.

_____ (1987), 'Agricultural growth linkages — the Bangladesh case', *Bangladesh Development Studies*, Vol. 15, No. 1, March.

_____ (1988), *Credit for Alleviation of Rural Poverty: The Grameen Bank in Bangladesh*. Research Report No. 65, International Food Policy Research Institute, Washington, D.C.

_____ (1990), 'Natural calamities, instability in production, and food policy in Bangladesh', *Bangladesh Development Studies*, Vol. 18, No. 1, March.

_____ and Asaduzzaman, M. (1983), 'An evaluation of special public works program in Bangladesh', *Bangladesh Development Studies*, Vol. 11, Nos. 1&2, March & June.

Hossain, Moazzem (1994), 'Alleviation of Food Poverty', in Zaffarullah, H.M. (ed.), *Policy Issues in Bangladesh*. New Delhi: South Asia Publishers.

Hossain, M. and Jones, S. (1983), 'Production, poverty, and the co-operative ideal: contradictions in Bangladesh rural development policy', in Lea, D. A. and Chaudhri, D.P., *Rural Development and the State*. London: Methuen.

Hunter, W.W. (1875), *A Statistical Account of Bengal*. London: Treubner and Co. (Reprinted in 1976 by Concept Publishing, Delhi)

Hussain, T. S. (1989), 'Economic development with and without land reform in Bangladesh', *Bangladesh Development Studies*, Vol. 17, No. 3, September.

ICMR (1951), *Results of Diet Surveys in India*. Hyderabad: Indian Council of Medical Research.

Ingram, J. (1988), 'The future of food aid', *Journal of World Food Program*, Nos. 6 and 7, April & September.

Iqbal, A. (1978), 'Unemployment and underemployment in Bangladesh agriculture', *World Development*, Vol. 6, Nos. 11 and 12, November & December.

IRRI (1977), *Constraints to High Yields on Asian Rice Farms*. Manila: IRRI.

IRRI (1981), *Annual Report* for 1981. Manila: IRRI.

———— (1993), *Rice in Crucial Environments*. Manila: IRRI.

Islam, I. and Khan, H. (1986), 'Income inequality, poverty, and socio-economic development in Bangladesh: an empirical investigation', *Bangladesh Development Studies*, Vol. 14, No. 2, June.

Islam, M.M. (1978), *Bengal Agriculture 1920-1946*. Cambridge: Cambridge University Press.

Islam, N. (1977), *Development Strategy of Bangladesh*. Oxford : Pergamon Press.

———— (1982), 'Food', in J. Faaland (ed). *Population and World Economy in the 21st Century*. Oxford: Basel Blackwell.

Ives, J. D. and Masserli, D. (1989), *The Himalayan Dilemma: Reconciling, Development, and Conservation*. London: Routledge.

Jackson, I.J. (1977), *Climate, Water, and Agriculture in the Tropics*. London: Longman.

Jain, S.C. (1986), 'Poverty alleviation programs in India: some issues of macro policy', *Indian Journal of Agricultural Economics*, Vol. 41, No. 3, July.

Jannuzi, F. T. and Peach, J. T. (1980), *Agrarian Structure in Bangladesh: a Constraint on Development*. Boulder: Westview Press.

Jansen, E. G. (1986), *Rural Bangladesh: Competition for Scarce Resources*. Oslo: Norwegian University Press.

Johnson, B. L. C. (1975), *Bangladesh*. London: Heinemann Educational Books.

Johnson, E.A.J. (1974), *The Organization of Space in Developing Countries*. Cambridge, Mass.: Harvard University Press.

Kakwani, N. (1989), 'On measuring undernutrition', *Oxford Economic Papers*, Vol.41, No. 4, March.

Kalirajan, K. P. and Shand, R. T. (1985), 'Types of education and agricultural productivity', *Journal of Development Studies*, Vol. 21, No. 2, January.

Kangle, R. P. (1965), *The Kautilya's Arthasastra*. Bombay: University of Bombay Press.

Kates, R. et al. (1988), *The Hunger Report: 1988*. Providence, R.I.: Brown University, World Hunger Program.

Kate, R. and Millman, S. (1990), 'On ending hunger: lessons from history', in Newman, L.F. (ed.), *Hunger in History*. Oxford: Basil Blackwell.

Kelly, K. (1981), 'Agricultural Change in Hoogly, 1850-1910', *Annals Association of American Geographers*, Vol. 71, No. 2, June.

Kennedy, E. T. and Cogill, B. (1987), *Income and Nutritional Effects of Commercialization of Agriculture in Southwestern Kenya.* Research Report No. 63, Washington, DC.: International Food Policy Research Institute.

Khan, A.R. (1977), 'Poverty and inequality in rural Bangladesh', in *Poverty and Landlessness in Rural Asia',* Geneva: ILO.

———— (1990), 'Poverty in Bangladesh: A consequence of and a constraint on growth', *Bangladesh Development Studies,* Vol. 18, No. 3, September.

———— and Hossain, M. (1989), *The Strategy of Development in Bangladesh.* London: Macmillan.

Khan, M. (1982), 'Rural urban migration and urbanizationin Bangladesh', *Geographical Review,* Vol.72, No. 4, October.

Khan, M. M. (1985), 'Labor absorption and unemployment in rural Bangladesh', *Bangladesh Development Studies,* Vol. 13, Nos. 3&4, September & December.

Khusro, A.M. (1964), 'Returns to scale in Indian Agriculture', *Indian Journal of Agricultural Economics,* Vol. 19, No. 1, January.

Klimkenborg, V. (1995), 'A farming revolution: sustainable agriculture', *National Geographic,* Vol. 188, No. 6, June.

Knight, J. B. and Sabot, R. H. (1987), 'Education policy and labor productivity: an output accounting exercise', *Economic Journal,* Vol. 97, No. !, March.

Kumar, B. G. (1985), *Poverty and Public Policy: Government Intervention and Levels of Living in Kerala, India.* Ph.D. Thesis, University of Oxford.

Lamptey, P. and Sai, F. T. (1985), 'Integrated health, nutrition, and population programs', in Biswas, M. and Pinstrup-Andersen, P. eds. *Nutrition and Development.* Oxford: Oxford University Press.

Lau, L. J. and P.A. Yotopoulos (1973), 'A test of relative efficiency and application to Indian agriculture', *American Economic Review,* Vol. 63, No. 1, March.

Lea, D.A. and Chaudhri, D.P. (1983), *Rural Development and the State.* London: Methuen.

Mahmud, W. (1990), 'Food supply and income distribution in a structuralist macro model', *Bangladesh Development Studies,* Vol. 18, No. 4, December.

Malthus, T. (1798), *First Essay on Population.* London: Macmillan. (Reprinted in 1966).

Maskina, M. S., Singh, B., and Singh, Y. (1987), 'Response of new rice varities to nitrogen', *International Rice Research Newsletter,* Vol. 12, No. 4, August.

Meadows, D. H. *et al.* (1972), *Limits to Growth.* London: Pan Books Ltd.

————(1992), *Beyond the Limits to Growth.* London: Earthscan Publications.

Mellor, J.W. and Stevens, R. D. (1965), 'The average and marginal product of farm labour', *Journal of Farm Economics,* Vol. 38, No. 2, March.

Mellor, J.W. (1988), 'Global Food Balances and food security', *World Development,* Vol. 16, No. 9, September.

Mellor, J.W. and Desai, G. (1985), *Agricultural Change and Rural Poverty.* Baltimore: Johns Hopkins Press.

Montgomery, R. (1985), 'Statutory rationing and modified rationing: causes and effects', *Bangladesh Development Studies*, Vol. 13, No. 1, March.

_____ (1985), 'Bangladesh floods of 1984 in historical context', *Disasters*, Vol. 9, No. 1, March.

Murshid, K. A. S. (1986), 'Instability in foodgrain production in Bangladesh: nature, levels, and trends', *Bangladesh Development Studies*, Vol. 15, No. 1, March.

Myrdal, G. (1977), *Asian Drama*. Harmondsworth: Penguin Books.

Narain, D. (1965), *Impact of Price Movements on Areas Under Selected Crops*, Cambridge: Cambridge University Press.

Oefhaf, R. C. (1978), *Organic Agriculture*. New York: John Wiley and Sons.

Osmani, S. R. (1990), 'Notes on some recent estimates of rural poverty in Bangladesh', *Bangladesh Development Studies*, Vol. 18, No. 3, September.

_____ (1991), 'Food Problems of Bangladesh', in Dreze, J. and Sen, Amartya (eds), *The Political Economy of Hunger*, Vol. 3. Oxford: Clarendon Press.

Osmani, S. R. (1989), 'Limits to the alleviation of poverty through non-farm credit', *Bangladesh Development Studies*, Vol. 17, No. 4, December.

Overbeek, J. (1976), *The Population Challenge*. London: Greenwood Press.

Pandey, P.C., Bisht, P. S., and Lal, P. (1995), 'Green manure: a substitute for inorganic fertilizers in lowland rice', *International Rice Research Notes*, Vol. 20, No. 1, March.

Piemental, D. (1984), 'Energy flow and the food systems', in Piemental, D. and Hall, C. W. (eds.), *Food and Energy Resources*. New York: Academic Press.

Pierce, J. T. (1990), *The Food Resources*. Harlow: Longman Scientific and Technical.

Pingali, P. L. and Binswanger, H. P. (1987), 'Population and agricultural intensification: a study of the evolution of technologies in tropical agriculture', in Johnson, D. G. and Lee, R. D. (eds.) *Population Growth and Economic Development: Issues and Evidence*. Madison: University of Wisconsin Press.

Pray, C. E. (1980), 'An assessment of the accuracy of official agricultural statistics of Bangladesh', *Bangladesh Development Studies*, Vol. 8, Nos. 1&2, March & June.

Quasem, A. (1987), 'Farmers participation in paddy markets, their marketed surplus, and factors affecting them in Bangladesh', *Bangladesh Development Studies*, Vol. 15, No. 1, March.

Rahaman, P. M. M. (1985), 'Poverty and inequality in land holding distribution in rural Bangladesh', *Indian Journal of Agricultural Economics*, Vol. 40, No. 4, October .

Rahman, A. (1979), 'Surplus utilization and capital formation in Bangladesh agriculture', *Bangladesh Development Studies*, Vol. 8, No. 4, September.

Rahman, A. (1987), 'Resource use in Bangladesh agriculture: an empirical analysis', *Bangladesh Development Studies* , Vol. 15, No. 1, March.

Rahman, A. and Haque, T. (1988), *Poverty and Inequality in Bangaladesh in the Eighties*. Research Report No. 91. Dhaka: Bangladesh Institute of Development Studies.

Rahman, S. H. (1986), 'Supply response in Bangladesh agriculture', *Bangladesh Development Studies*, Vol. 14, No. 1, March.

Rao, C.H. (1972), 'Uncertainty, entrepreneurship, and sharecropping in India', *Journal of Political Economy*, Vol. 79, No. 3, May & June.

Rao, V. and Chotigeat, T. (1981), 'Inverse relationship between size of land holdings and agricultural productivity', *American Journal of Agricultural Economics*, Vol. 63, No. 3, August.

Rao, V. K. R. V. (1982), *Food, Nutrition, and Poverty in India.* Delhi: Vikas Publication.

Raup, P.M. (1982), 'An agricultural critique of the national agricultural land study', *Land Economics*, Vol. 58, No. 2, May.

Ravallian, M. (1982), 'Agricultural wages in Bangladesh before and after 1974 famine', *Bangladesh Development Studies*, Vol. 10, No. 1, March.

_____ (1990), 'Arithmatic of poverty in Bangladesh', *Bangladesh Development Studies*, Vol. 18, No. 3, September.

Raychaudhuri, T. (1953), *Bengal Under Akbar and Jhangir.* Delhi: Munshiram and Mohanlal.

Raznov, B. *et al.* (1990), 'Soils', in Turner, B.L. *et al.* (eds), *The Earth as Transformed by Human Action.* Cambridge : Cambridge University Press.

Ricardo, D. (1987 Reprint), *The Principles of Political Ecopnomy.* Dent: London.

Rizvi, N. (1987), 'Socio-cultural chain and family food availability in Bangladesh', in UNESCO, *Food Deficiency: Studies and Perspectives.* Bangkok: UNESCO.

Robinson, C.H. (1978), *Fundamentals of Normal Nutrition.* New York: Macmillan Publishing Company.

Robinson, W. and Schutjer, W. (1984), 'Agricultural development and demographic generalization of Boserup's model', *Economic Development and Cultural Change*, Vol. 62, No. 2, January.

Rosegrant, M. W. and Svendsen, M. (1993), 'Asian food production in the 1990s', *Food Policy*, Vol. 18, No. 1, February.

Ryot, A. (1858), *Indigo Cultivation in Bengal.* Calcutta: Stanhope Press.

Salma, U. and Warr, P. G. (1994), *Foodgrain Policy in Bangladesh.* Canberra: National Centre for Development.

Schultz, T. W. (1964), *Transforming Traditional Agriculture.* New Haven: Yale Univeristy.

Sen, A. (1960), *Choice of Techniques.* Oxford: Blackwell.

_____ (1964), 'Size of holding and productivity', *Economic Weekly* , Vol. 16, Nos. 5-7 (Annual Number), February.

_____ (1981), *Poverty and Famine.* Oxford: Oxford University Press.

_____ (1984), *Resources, Values, and Development.* Oxford: Basil Blackwell.

Shahabuddin, Q. (1989), 'Pattern of food consumption in Bangladesh', *Bangladesh Development Studies*, Vol. 17, No. 3, September.

Simon, J. (1977), *The Economics of Population Growth*. Princeton: Princeton University Press.

———— (1975), 'The positive effect of population growth on agricultural saving in irrigation systems'. *Review of Economics and Statistics*, Vol. 57, No. 1, Feburary.

———— (1981), *The Ultimate Resource*, Oxford: Martin Robertson and Co.

———— (1983), 'Effects of population on nutrition and well-being', in Rotberg, R. I. and Rabb, T. K., *Hunger and History*. Cambridge: Cambridge University Press.

Singh, B. (1947), *Population Planning in India*. Bombay: Asia Publishing House.

Singh, J. P. (1975), 'Resource use, farm size, and return to scale in a backward agriculture', *Indian Journal of Agricultural Economics*, Vol. 30, No. 2, April.

Singh, I. (1988), *Small Farms in South Asia: Their Characteristics, Productivity, and Efficiency*. Washington, D.C.: World Bank.

———— (1990), *The Great Ascent: The Rural Poor in South Asia*. Baltimore: Johns Hopkins University Press.

Smith, W. E. (1988), 'A country under water', *Time*, September 19.

Sobhan, R. (1990), ' The politics of hunger and entitlement', in J. Dereze and Sen, A. (eds.), *Political Economy of Hunger*. Vol 1. Oxford: Oxford University Press.

Spate, O.H.K. and Learmonth, A.T.A. (1967), *India and Pakistan*. London: Methuen.

Srinivasan, T. (1983), 'Measuring malnutrition', *Ceres*, Vol. 16, No. 1, March.

Stamp, E. (1977), *Growing Out of Poverty*. Oxford: Oxford University Press.

Stevens, R. D. and Jabara, C. L. (1988), *Agricultural Development Principles: Economic Theory and Empirical Evidence*. Baltimore: Johns Hopkins Press.

Subramanian, V. (1975), *Parched Earth: The Maharashtra Drought*. Bombay: Orient Longmans.

Subramaniyan, G. and Nirmala, V. (1991), 'A macro analysis of fertilizer demand in India', *Indian Journal of Agricultural Economics* , Vol. 46, No. 1, January.

Sudhir, A. and Kanbur, S. M. R. (1991), 'Public policy and basic needs provision: interventions and achievement in Shri Lanka', in Dereze, J. and Sen, A. (eds.), *The Political Economy of Hunger, Vol. 3*. Oxford: Clarendon Press.

Sukhatme, P.V. (1977), 'Incidence of undernutriton', *Indian Journal of Agricultural Economics*, Vol. 32, No. 1, January.

———— (1978), 'Assessment of adequacy of diet at different income levels', *Economic and Political Weekly*, Vol. 13, Nos. 31-33, August.

———— (1981), 'On measurement of poverty', *Economic and Political Weekly*, Vol. 32, No. 24, June.

———— and Margen, S. (1982), 'Autoregulatory homeostatic nature of energy balance', *American Journal of Clinical Nutrition*, Vol. 35, No. 2, February.

Tabah, L. (1982), 'Population growth', in Faaland, J. (ed.) *Population and World Economy in the 21 Century*. Oxford: Basil Blackwell.

Tarrant, J. R. (1982), 'Food policy conflicts in Bangladesh', *World Development*, Vol. 10, No. 2, February.

Taslim, M. A. (1989), 'Supervision problem and size productivity relation in Bangladesh argiculture', *Oxford Bulletin of Economics and Statistics*, Vol. 51, No.1, February.

Thompson, P. B. (1992), *The Ethics of Aid and Trade*. Cambridge: Cambridge University Press.

Turner II, B. L *et al.* (1977), 'Population pressure and agrucultural intensity', *Annals of the Association of American Geographers*, Vol. 67, No. 3, September.

_____ (1989), 'The specialist-synthesis approach to the revival of geography: The case of cultural ecology', *Annals Association of American Geographers* , Vol. 79, No. 1, March.

_____ (1990), *The Earth as Transformed by Human Action*. Cambridge: Cambridge University Press.

_____ and Kates, R. (1990), 'The great transformation', in Turner, B.L. et al. *The Earth as Transformed by Human Action*. Cambridge: Cambridge University Press.

Umitsu, M. (1993), 'Late quaternary sedimentary environments and landforms in Ganges Delta', *Sedimentary Geology*, Vol. 83, No. 2, March.

UNICEF (1995), *State of the World's Children: 1995*. Oxford: Oxford University Press.

Uvin, P. (1994), *The International Organization of Hunger*. London: Kegan and Paul.

Warnock, J.W. (1987), *The Politics of Hunger*. London: Methuen.

Weaver, J. C. (1954), 'Changing pattern of cropland use in the Middle-West', *Economic Geography*, Vol. 30, No. 1, January.

_____ (1954), 'Crop combination regions in the Middle-West', *The Geographical Review*, Vol. 44, No. 1, January.

Whittlow, J. (1980), *Disasters*. London: Penguin Books.

World Bank (1986), *Bangladesh*. Oxford: Oxford University Press.

_____ (1990), *World Development Report*. Oxford: Oxford University Press.

Yotopoulos, P.A. and Lau, L.J. (1973), 'A test of relative economic efficiency: some further results', *American Economic Journal*, Vol. 63, No. 1, March.

Index